HANDBOOK

OUTPATIENT PARENTERAL ANTIMICROBIAL THERAPY

For Infectious Diseases

ALAN D. TICE, MD, FACP

CRG PUBLISHING

A DIVISION OF THE CURRY ROCKEFELLER GROUP, LLC

Publication of this handbook is sponsored by AAF-MED LLC, 660 White Plains Road, Suite 535, Tarrytown, New York 10591, and supported by an educational grant from Cubist Pharmaceuticals, Inc., 65 Hayden Avenue, Lexington, Massachusetts 02426. The opinions expressed represent the views of the author and should not be construed to represent the opinions of the provider, publisher, or any commercial supporters.

HANDBOOK *of*
OUTPATIENT PARENTERAL ANTIMICROBIAL THERAPY
For Infectious Diseases

by ALAN D. TICE, MD, FACP

Associate Professor
University of Hawaii at Manoa
John A. Burns School of Medicine
Honolulu, Hawaii

CONTRIBUTING EDITORS

Nancy Mortlock, *RN, CRNI, OCN, Director of Clinical Services, US Oncology, Cancer Care Northwest, Tacoma, Washington;* V. James Fiorenzo, *RPh, MBA, Senior Vice President, Strategic and Support Services, President, Regional Health Services, Inc., HAMOT Health Foundation, Erie, Pennsylvania;* Robert E. Buzas, *RPh, Director of Pharmacy, Great Lakes Home Healthcare, Erie, Pennsylvania;* Sheri Karanasos, *Editor, OPAT Sourcebook, Tacoma, Washington;* Barbara Ross Nolet, *RN, MA, ARNP/MS, Northwest Management, Gig Harbor, Washington*

CRG PUBLISHING, A DIVISION OF THE CURRY ROCKEFELLER GROUP, LLC

Library of Congress Control Number 2006929707

Publishing Director	Linnéa C. Elliott
Project Editor	Jean O'Hara Fitzpatrick
Senior Editor	Bridget Maron
Program Coordinator	Eileen Hernández
CME Provider	AAF-MED, LLC
Composition	DM Cradle Associates
Printing	Commercial Offset

ISBN: 0-9786457-0-7

The Curry Rockefeller Group, LLC, 660 White Plains Road, Tarrytown, New York 10591

Contents

Preface

■ *Accreditation and Designation of Credit*

AAF-MED is accredited by the Accreditation Council for Continuing Medical Education (ACCME) to provide continuing medical education for physicians.

AAF-MED designates this educational activity for a maximum of 4 *AMA PRA Category 1 Credits™*. Physicians should only claim credit commensurate with the extent of their participation in the activity.

Nonphysician participants claiming credit will receive a certificate of participation.

■ *Release Date*

September 1, 2006

■ *Termination Date*

August 31, 2007

This CME activity has been planned and produced in accordance with the ACCME Essentials and Standards for Commercial Support.

This enduring material will be reviewed within 1 year of its release date and rereleased, or its designation for CME credit will become invalid on its expiration date.

■ *Statement of Need*

The practice of administering outpatient parenteral antimicrobial therapy (OPAT) in the home and in other community settings has grown rapidly over the past 20 years, reflecting the dramatic progress in clinical, pharmaceutical, and technological research. The current emphasis on cost control and managed care has also created a powerful impetus to move and keep some patients out of high-cost hospital beds for therapeutic interventions traditionally delivered in hospitals. It is estimated that more then 250,000 Americans are treated with OPAT each year, with its growth rate estimated to exceed 10% annually. The educational goal of the *Handbook of Outpatient Parenteral Antimicrobial Therapy* is to provide the latest data regarding the delivery, efficacy, safety, and future of OPAT to the physicians, nurses, pharmacists, social workers, and ancillary health care professionals who make up the OPAT team. The Handbook is also designed to introduce physicians to OPAT as a potential therapeutic option for their patients.

■ *Target Audience*

Current OPAT teams, infectious disease specialists, primary care physicians, emergency room physicians, visiting nurses, infusion nurses, pharmacists, and health care personnel involved with home care.

■ *Learning Objectives*

On completion of the *Handbook of Outpatient Parenteral Antimicrobial Therapy*, readers should be able to:

- Identify patient candidates for OPAT from those presenting in the office or those already hospitalized
- Name the infections amenable to OPAT
- List the antimicrobial(s) appropriate to treating specific diseases with OPAT
- Define the most appropriate intravenous catheter for antimicrobial delivery according to individual patient situations and preferences
- Appraise whether a port should be placed, depending on the patient's condition, treatment situation, and preference; be able to choose the port that is most appropriate
- Describe the infusion device best suited to the patient's treatment requirements and preference
- Detail a quality measurement program based on clinical outcomes as well as program structure and process

- As a referring physician, define an OPAT program that will fulfill an individual patient's needs for safe, effective, quality care
- Recognize the legal issues associated with OPAT
- Evaluate reimbursement from Medicare, Medicaid, Blue Cross/Blue Shield

■ *Faculty Disclosure*

Individuals who are in a position to control the content of a CME activity must disclose to the learners all relevant financial relationships with any commercial interest providing products or services that may be related to the content of the continuing medical education activity.

Alan D. Tice, MD, FACP, reports the following relationships with commercial interests: grants/research support: Schering-Plough Corp., F. Hoffmann-La Roche Ltd., Cubist Pharmaceuticals, Inc., Merck & Co., Inc.; consultant, speakers bureau: Merck & Co., Inc., Cubist Pharmaceuticals, Inc.; advisory board member: Merck & Co., Inc., Pfizer Inc.

Nancy Mortlock, RN, CNRI, OCN, reports she has no commercial relationships to disclose with regard to this activity.

V. James Fiorenzo, RPh, MBA, reports he has no commercial relationships to disclose with regard to this activity.

Robert E. Buzas, RPh, reports he has no commercial relationships to disclose with regard to this activity.

Sheri Karanasos reports she has no commercial relationships to disclose with regard to this activity.

Barbara Ross Nolet, RN, MA, ARNP/MS, reports the following relationships with commercial interests: consultant, speakers bureau: Roche Laboratories, Cubist Pharmaceuticals, Inc.

Acknowledgements

The course of OPAT has been a challenging one, particularly from a physician standpoint. It is my hope that this handbook will bring some knowledge and encouragement to physicians and the nurses, pharmacists, administrators, and others who work with them to develop even better care for people who can benefit from outpatient care for serious infections.

In looking back over the time and energy spent in the efforts to bring this handbook to press for the community of infectious diseases specialists and their teams, I would like to thank my wife, Constance, and my daughter, Amanda, for their patience and support over the years. I would also like to thank my former partners and the staff of Infections Limited for their insight and understanding.

In addition, I would like you to know that Barbara Ross Nolet and Nancy Mortlock have made major contributions to many of the chapters in this handbook and that it would not have been possible without them. Sheri Karanasos, Robert Buzas, and James Fiorenzo have also been most helpful with their contributions and reviews.

I thank you all for your interest in OPAT and hope the information contained within will be of value in improving the care you can provide for your patients in the outpatient setting.

Alan D. Tice, MD, FACP

Introduction

The growth of programs that offer intravenous (IV) infusion therapy outside the hospital setting reflects the dramatic progress in clinical, pharmaceutical, and technological research. The resulting development of new drugs and IV infusion devices led to improvements in the delivery of outpatient care and in patient satisfaction. The current emphasis on cost control and managed care has also created a powerful impetus to move or keep some patients out of high-cost hospital beds for therapeutic interventions traditionally delivered in hospitals.

Outpatient parenteral antimicrobial therapy (OPAT) for infectious disease was first described in the United States in 1974[1] and has grown into an industry that generates revenues of more than a billion dollars annually.[2] Drug infusion therapy, most often delivered intravenously but subcutaneously and intrathecally as well, continues to grow with the expansion of home health care.[3]

The program at Infections Limited was initiated 23 years ago to treat patients who were participating in clinical trials of ceftriaxone, a third-generation cephalosporin with prolonged serum activity requiring only one dose a day. It became difficult to justify these patients' hospitalization, so outpatient infusion was begun as an extension of the office practice.[4,5] Many OPAT programs were begun for similar reasons of cost savings and patient convenience.

The following chapters describe the available models of OPAT, the development and implementation of home care plans, and the current opportunities and challenges offered by this relatively new concept of medical care. A brief overview of OPAT's proven and potential contributions to the improvement of clinical care and outcome in patients with infectious diseases as well as the problems inherent in this change of clinical venue may be helpful.

■ *Patient Benefits*

Patients treated outside the hospital, whether in an outpatient facility or at home, avoid problems inherent in the hospital system, including unfamiliar, sometimes frightening surroundings; isolation from friends and family; lack of privacy; and increased risk of secondary infections. With OPAT, patients can recover in the comfort of their own homes, and many can return to work or school. Avoiding or leaving the hospital setting also may facilitate the transition from the role of sick "patient" back to the familiar, functioning self, thus speeding both adaptation and recovery.[6-8]

In OPAT programs, treatment is adjusted to each patient's lifestyle. One of the important questions asked of candidates for the program is "What is your usual day like?" Then, on the basis of the answers, the feasibility of OPAT, the most appropriate delivery system, and the least obtrusive dosing schedule can be determined.

Children are at a particular disadvantage when it comes to hospitalization. They are less adaptable than most adults to unfamiliar surroundings and have little understanding of their illness and the often threatening and painful procedures involved. The incidence of nosocomial infections in children is proportional to their age, with the highest incidence occurring in neonates and children one year of age.[9] Early discharge to outpatient care as soon as their condition is stable is particularly desirable for children. The success of this approach has resulted in consideration of OPAT without initial hospitalization for children who don't require skilled nursing observation during the first hours of therapy.

The fact that most people prefer being treated at home rather than in the hospital is repeatedly demonstrated by a post-therapy patient satisfaction survey administered at Infections Limited. When asked whether they would prefer outpatient or hospital treatment for any future illness requiring IV therapy, 95% of patients say they would opt for outpatient care again.[10] Similar results have been reported by other outpatient providers.[11-13]

Successful OPAT requires patients' participation as well as some level of responsibility for their own treatment program. To this end, patients and caregivers must be informed about their disease or infection; the therapeutic intervention, including handling and maintenance of the delivery system; and the problems to look for. The resulting knowledge and sense of control can facilitate recovery and, for some patients, can decrease pain and side effects. The patients who learn to self-administer IV antimicrobials often take great pride in the skills they have acquired and are delighted when given a certificate of accomplishment at the end of therapy.

■ *Health Care-Related Infections*

Hospital-related infections have been estimated to affect over 5% of hospitalized patients, with an average 4-day extension of hospitalization and a direct loss of more than 20,000 lives annually in the United States.[14-17] According to the Centers for Disease Control and Prevention's (CDC's) National Nosocomial Infections Surveillance (NNIS) system, which receives monthly reports of nosocomial infections from more than 270 hospitals in the United States, the infection rate has remained remarkably stable over the years, with approximately 5 to 6 hospital-acquired infections for every 100 admissions.[18] However, because of progressively shorter hospital stays, the rate of such infections per 1,000 patient days actually increased from 7.2 in 1975 to 9.8 in 1995, a 36% growth. As of 1995, these infections cost $4.5 billion and have contributed to more than 88,000 deaths, one death every 6 minutes. Moreover these numbers have grown with each passing year. Additional health care costs in excess of $10 billion annually have been estimated as a result of nosocomial bloodstream infections alone,[19] which account for 8% of all hospital-related infections reported in the United States.[20]

Although the risk of infection directly related to outpatient IV therapy has not been quantified, the incidence appears to be far less than that related to hospitalization.[21] The phlebitis rate associated with IV antimicrobials is also greater in hospitalized patients than in those treated at home according to some reports.[13]

Another problem in the hospital setting is the increased prevalence of organisms that are highly resistant to the antimicrobials used against community-acquired infections. Multidrug-resistant staphylococci, enterococci, and gram-negative bacteria typically lurk in hospitals. Infections related to outpatient therapy have not yet been given a descriptive name. However, the term "nosohusial" (Greek "nosos" for disease and Old English "hus" for house) has been proposed.[21]

■ Cost Containment

A number of studies have documented the cost savings of OPAT.[22-24] A hospital bed often costs more than $1,000 a day in the United States, with the fixed overhead costs of maintaining the physical plant, purchase and maintenance of equipment, provision of meals, and nursing and administrative staff.[25] As the health care system continues its dramatic shift away from costly and often prolonged hospital care, models of advanced medical care outside the hospital setting continue to improve. Many can deliver comparable—even higher—quality care at less cost than that possible in hospitals. In the self-administration model of OPAT home infusion, for example, patients or family members administer IV medications at home, thereby eliminating overhead and staff cost.

The comparative economics of hospital and outpatient IV antimicrobial therapy must take into account the rather different objectives associated with the two therapeutic settings. In the hospital, all efforts are directed toward curing patients and discharging them, with an eye to maximizing profit and minimizing loss.[23,24] Cure of an infection is also the objective of outpatient IV antimicrobial therapy, but outside the circumscribed hospital setting, the patient's quality of life becomes a significant concern that must be factored, with outcome, into the cost-benefit analysis.

■ OPAT Outcomes and Quality Assurance

The measurement of outcomes by an OPAT program is a part of the continuous performance improvement process through which health care providers attempt to improve and ensure the quality of their care and services. Quality assurance activities required or recommended by accrediting and licensing bodies have generally focused on the presence of administrative and patient care procedures as indicators of quality, rather than actual clinical outcome. Moreover, the best-studied OPAT outcomes indicators have been those related to cost savings and financial analyses.[25] As the financial pressures mount for earlier hospital discharge of sicker patients, the importance of monitoring outcomes to ensure patient safety increases. Accrediting bodies such as the Joint Commission for the Accreditation of Healthcare Organizations (JCAHO) and the National Committee for Quality Assurance (NCQA) require outcomes measurements as a part of their certification process but do not specify the parameters or indicators to use. Not only have we lacked an adequate system for collection of reliable data to assess the clinical aspects of programs, but there is as yet no consensus as to what those data should be.

Thus, despite its success, OPAT—indeed, the entire field of outpatient care—has, until recently, been without accepted standard-of-care guidelines (see Chapter 7). A system for outcome measures with OPAT has been proposed that takes into account clinical and bacterial outcomes as well as physician evaluations.[26] The 2004 Practice Guidelines for Outpatient Parenteral Antimicrobial Therapy,[26] formulated from the collective experience of the OPAT Outcomes Registry,[27] as well as several major OPAT programs across the United States, describe the important aspects of OPAT. Outcomes measures are included as an integral part of the OPAT program to ensure both its effectiveness and quality of care.

■ *Reimbursement*

Third-party payment for OPAT, like that for all health care, is regulated by a multitude of private and public health policies (see Chapter 8). Outpatient IV infusion therapy is currently viewed by many third-party payers as outpatient therapy per se rather than as a lower-cost alternative to hospitalization. Physicians are not usually reimbursed for their services without seeing the patient. Physician case management services have not been compensated for OPAT. Although Medicare now allows payments to physicians for office infusions, they are specifically excluded unless a physician is physically present. The question of reimbursement continues to undergo rapid changes with the growth of managed care and the passage of health care legislation.

■ *Medicolegal Issues*

Legal responsibility and liability for outpatient care is a major concern that involves issues of quality assurance and cost containment. The limitations of patient safety have not been defined in home care yet the financial pressures are tremendous and growing for early discharge. Litigation in home care is increasing (see Chapter 9).

In most courts, the legal and ultimate responsibility for quality of outpatient therapy rests with the physician as "captain of the ship," with the standard of care to which he or she is held for patients receiving OPAT comparable to that expected in the hospital. Moreover, the law regarding physician ownership of or financial involvement with companies to which they might refer patients remains vague enough to raise complex legal issues of self-referral and kickbacks. The situation will continue to change as advances in appropriate therapeutic agents and delivery systems allow sicker patients to be discharged from the hospital or to avoid hospitalization altogether.

■ *Problems*

Although the success of outpatient IV infusion of antimicrobials has been remarkable in terms of efficacy, safety, cost savings, and patient satisfaction, its limits are uncertain and, in large part, unknown. The problems associated with outpatient therapy are different from those found in the hospital, where emergency staff and equipment are readily available. There is much less medical supervision and control of the patient's environment at home, particularly with the reduced number of physician visits and lack of compensation for their services. Home health care agencies conduct home visits to determine the safety of the environment before accepting patients. If safety of a home is in question, an alternative plan, such as treatment at an ambulatory clinic, may be required.

Outpatient therapy also puts patients at greater risk should severe reactions to medication or rapid deterioration of a disease state occur at home. Because of possible emergencies, many OPAT programs will not accept patients who do not have a telephone and ready access to transportation or ambulance services.

■ *The Future*

Although the challenges of OPAT are many, its rewards in terms of benefits to patients and their families, as well as potential cost savings, are great. Its future lies with the interest and creativity and energy of the physicians, nurses, pharmacists, and health care professionals who provide OPAT in each community.

References

1. Rucker RW, Harrison GM. Outpatient intravenous medications in the management of cystic fibrosis. *Pediatrics.* 1974;54:358–360.

2. Winters RW. The home infusion therapy industry: an overview. In: Conners RB, Winters RW, eds. *Home Infusion: Current Status and Future Trends.* Chicago, IL: American Hospitals Publishing Company; 1995:1–15.

3. Congress of the United States, Office of Technology Assessment. Chapter 4. The home drug infusion industry. In: *Home Drug Infusion Therapy Under Medicare.* Washington, DC: U.S. Government Printing Office; 1992:71–83.

4. Tice AD. Once-daily ceftriaxone outpatient therapy in adults with infections. *Chemotherapy.* 1991;37(suppl 3):7–10.

5. Tice AD. An office model of outpatient parenteral antibiotic therapy. *Rev Infect Dis.* 1991;13(suppl 2):S184–188.

6. Fawcett J. Orem's self-care model. In: Fawcett J, ed. *Analysis and Evaluation of Conceptual Models of Nursing*. Philadelphia, PA: F.A. Davis Company; 1984.

7. Fine MJ, Pratt HM, Obrosky DS, et al. Relation between length of hospital stay and costs of care for patients with community-acquired pneumonia. *Am J Med*. 2000;109:378–385.

8. Eron LJ, Passos S. Early discharge of infected patients through appropriate antibiotic use. *Arch Intern Med*. 2001;161:61–65.

9. MacQueen S. The special needs of children receiving intravenous therapy. *Nurs Times*. 2005;101:59, 61–62, 64.

10. Tice AD. Physician-directed, clinic-based program for outpatient intravenous antibiotic therapy. In: Conners RB, Winters RW, eds. *Home Infusion: Current Status and Future Trends*. Chicago, IL: American Hospital Publishing Company; 1995:103–114.

11. Cochrane S. A mark of approval. Patient satisfaction with an IV self-infusion teaching programme. *Prof Nurse*. 1994;10:106–111.

12. Huminer D, Pitlik S. Home IV antibiotic therapy in Israel [abstract]. *Intl Cong Infect Dis*. 1994;97.

13. Stiver G, Wai AO, Chase L, et al. Outpatient intravenous antibiotic therapy: the Vancouver Hospital experience. *Can J Infect Dis*. 2000;11(suppl A):11a–14a.

14. Brachman PS. Nosocomial infection control: an overview. *Rev Infect Dis*. 1981;3:640–648.

15. Dixon RE. Effect of infections on hospital care. *Ann Intern Med*. 1978;89(suppl):749–753.

16. Jorup Ronstrom C, Britton S. The nosocomial component of medical care. A prospective study on the amount, spectrum and costs of medical disturbances in a department of infectious diseases. *Scand J Infect Dis*. 1982;36(suppl):150–156.

17. McGowan JE Jr. Cost and benefit in control of nosocomial infection: methods for analysis. *Rev Infect Dis*. 1981;3:790–797.

18. Weinstein RA. Nosocomial infection update. *Emerg Infect Dis*. 1998;4:416–420. Available at: www.cdc.gov/ncidod/eid/vol4no3/weinstein.htm. Accessed June 21, 2006.

19. Edmond MB, Wenzel RP. Organization for infection control. In: Mandell G, Bennett JE, Dolin R, eds. *Principles and Practice of Infectious Diseases*. 6th ed. Philadelphia, PA: Churchill Livingstone; 2004:3323–3326.

20. Gura KM. Incidence and nature of epidemic nosocomial infections. *J Infus Nurs*. 2004;27:175–180.

21. Graham DR. Nosohusial infections: complications of home infusion therapy. *Infect Dis Clin Pract*. 1993;2:158–161.

22. Tice AD, Hoaglund PA, Nolet B, et al. Cost perspectives for outpatient intravenous antimicrobial therapy. *Pharmacotherapy* 2002;22(pt 2):63S–70S.

23. Milkovich G. Benefits of outpatient parenteral antibiotic therapy: to the individual, the institution, third party payers and society. *Int J Antimicrob Agents*. 1995;5:27–31.

24. A day in the hospital (updated 7/28/04). *The Ultimate Field Guide to the U.S. Economy*. Available at: www.fguide.org. Accessed May 17, 2005.

25. Tice AD. Pharmacoeconomic considerations in the ambulatory use of parenteral cephalosporins. *Drugs*. 2000;59(suppl 3):29–35.

26. Tice AD, Rehm SJ, Dalovisio JR, et al. Practice guidelines for outpatient parenteral antimicrobial therapy. ISDA guidelines. *Clin Infect Dis*. 2004;38:1651–1672.

27. Nathwani D, Tice A. Ambulatory antimicrobial use: the value of an outcomes registry. *J Antimicrob Chemother*. 2002;49:149–154.

CHAPTER 1

An Overview of Outpatient Parenteral Antimicrobial Therapy

Outpatient parenteral antimicrobial therapy (OPAT) can be delivered in almost any setting. Most programs are unique because their formats are dictated by local needs and resources. During the past few years, however, experience has resulted in increasing standardization and consolidation into three basic models of OPAT delivery:[1,2] at an infusion center; at home, administered by a nurse infusion specialist; and at home, administered by the patient or caregiver (Figure 1.1). Although not discussed here, the nursing home or convalescent center may be included as a fourth model. Each model has both clinical and economic advantages and disadvantages (Table 1.1).[3]

■ *The Infusion Center Model*

An infusion center may be developed in a variety of medical settings, including a physician's office, a hospital clinic, an urgent care center, an emergency department (ED), or an independent facility. Regardless of setting, such centers function essentially as day hospitals, offering most of the equipment, facilities, and medical staff available in the hospital.

The infusion center model represents a good way to extend hospital-level care into the outpatient setting, with staffing, equipment, and physician involvement similar to that of the inpatient setting. The change from hospital to outpatient facility is less drastic than going directly to home care and may therefore be more acceptable to both medical personnel and patients. A successful program can be

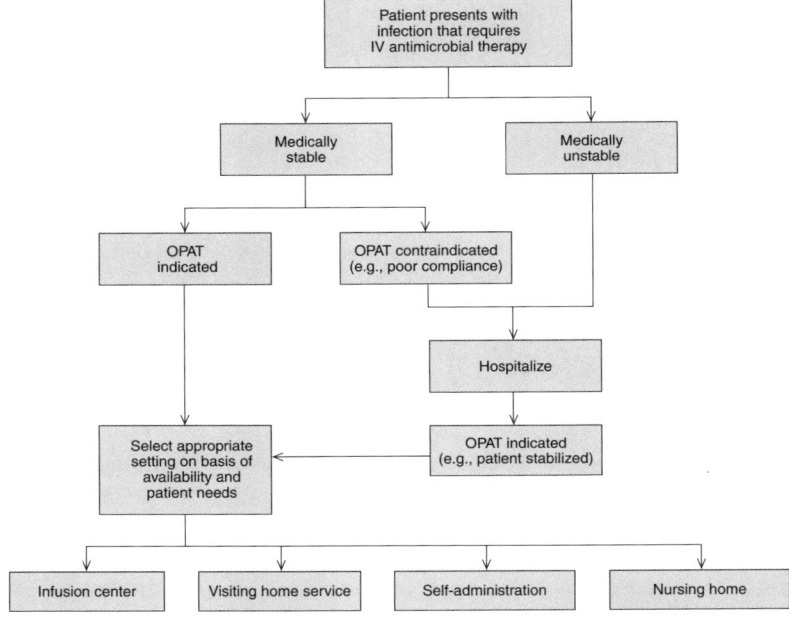

Figure 1.1. *Models of OPAT Delivery.*

expanded to include home infusion as well, administered by a nurse specialist, the patient, or a caregiver.

One limitation of the infusion center model is the difficulty of treating patients who need parenteral therapy more than once a day. This puts a premium on drugs that can be given once daily or on pumps that can be programmed to administer antimicrobials over a 24-hour period (see Chapter 4). Patients who have trouble walking or who lack transportation also may limit the use of infusion centers.

The Doctor's Office

The expansion of a physician's practice to include OPAT offers the advantage of close physician management and supervision with quick, appropriate treatment of problems and modifications in therapy. The office-based center is often more accessible to patients than the hospital clinic.[4] This model also allows the physician to have more control over the quality of OPAT services and responsiveness.

Table 1.1.   Pros and Cons of OPAT Delivery Models

Model	Advantages	Disadvantages
Infusion center	Medical staff on hand Access to medications and devices Supervised administration Physician available	Cost of facility Patient travel
Visiting nurse	Inspection of home Supervised administration	Cost of nurse time and travel Privacy concerns
Self-administration	Reduced costs Patient autonomy	Unsupervised administration Compliance Patient training
Nursing home	Medical staff Access to medications and devices Supervised administration Can deal with dementia and drug abuse	Cost of facility Staff training

Reprinted from Tice et al,[3] with permission.

The Hospital-Based Infusion Center

Much of today's OPAT is administered through hospital-based home care programs. A program may be organized as a division of the institution or as a separate affiliated entity. In the first situation, the hospital pharmacy provides medication and equipment and the nursing staff delivers care. The independent affiliate has its own pharmacy, nursing, equipment, management, and delivery services separate from and outside the hospital.

Another hospital-based option is incorporation of OPAT into established clinics or day hospitals. Patients can be scheduled during slow times at a walk-in clinic. The cost of building or leasing and maintaining a new facility can thereby be avoided. The costs of equipment depreciation and, if necessary, additional staffing are negligible compared with those of hospital care providing around-the-clock staffing, food, and other inpatient care.

The Hospital Emergency Department

Emergency departments may also serve as infusion centers, with administration of single daily doses of parenteral antibiotics and successive evaluation of patients until therapy is completed or clinical response is adequate to justify a switch to oral agents. Infusion therapy may be scheduled rather than being random or urgent, and can be administered during the ED's slow hours.[5] Some ED infusion centers have incorporated observation units, allowing the initiation of parenteral treatment under skilled supervision, while freeing up ED beds for new patients.

■ *The Visiting Nurse Model*

In this model, a nurse specialist trained in intravenous (IV) therapy travels to the patient's home to administer an injection or IV infusion. Patients who have limited mobility, are bedridden, or are difficult to transport may require treatment at home. For those with a terminal malignancy or with advanced AIDS, such visits may allow patients to spend their remaining lives in the comfort and privacy of their own homes in the care of family and friends.

A major advantage of home-based infusion is that it allows the nurse to evaluate the home situation for factors often overlooked in the hospital.[6] He or she can assess physical limitations, environmental hazards, and domestic issues, as well as drug or alcohol abuse that would affect a patient's therapy or response. Additional skilled services, such as physical therapy, occupational therapy, and social services, can be provided in the home as well.

A limiting factor in this model may be the cost of the nurse specialist's time and travel. In some urban settings, one nurse can easily visit 5 to 10 patients in one working day, whereas in rural areas, travel time may make the cost of this model prohibitive. If a nurse must drive an hour to visit a patient, continued hospitalization may be more reasonable. Also, for an antimicrobial that requires multiple doses per day, the cost advantage of nurse administration may be lost and other models should be considered.

Other problems that are associated with the visiting nurse model include the concern with privacy felt by some patients and the possible threat to nurses' safety posed by some neighborhoods.

■ *The Self-Administration Model*

The concept of patient self-administration of OPAT grew out of successful experience in training patients and their families to provide long-term total parenteral nutrition at home.[7] Many patients were even taught to mix their own solutions. Patients with immunoglobulin deficiency and hemophilia have also been trained in self-administration,[8] as have patients with AIDS who have complicating fungal or viral infections.[9] The days- to weeks-long courses of IV antibiotics required for severe infections are now being administered by many patients themselves, particularly those who feel otherwise well enough to return to work or school. However, given recent changes in pharmacy practice, it is no longer acceptable for patients to mix their own infusion medications, except for those which, because of high cost or short shelf life, cannot be mixed in an infusion pharmacy clean room.

For children or patients with physical or mental limitations that preclude self-administration, a parent, spouse, or other caregiver often can be trained in the techniques of OPAT administration and venous access device care.[10] In fact, it is often wise to train one or more people in addition to the patient to provide backup if it is needed.

Patients are often overlooked as valuable human resources in health care. Most are remarkably adept when it comes to their own care. They can be taught the techniques of IV therapy within a few hours and, with the right backup and support, can become quite expert. One study found fewer IV line problems in a group of patients who administered their own OPAT than in a group treated in the hospital.[11]

The self-administration model offers considerable financial savings, particularly for prolonged courses of treatment, afforded by essentially eliminating personnel and overhead costs. As a result of dramatic decreases in reimbursement by the insurance industry, home infusion companies can no longer afford to send nurses to homes to perform infusions. Thus the role of the home care nurse as well as the pharmacist is now that of clinical educator, to instruct patient and caregiver on the many aspects of appropriate infusion therapy. An infusion facility may still be needed, however, to provide initial doses of antimicrobials and vascular access, patient training, and pharmacy services, as well as medical supervision.

Patients or caregivers who administer medication need consistent support and monitoring to ensure compliance and patient response. Telephone communication between home and infusion facility is crucial, with periodic calls from a health care professional to check on patient status and any incipient or actual problems. Patient visits to an infusion facility or nurse visits to the patient's home may still be needed on an intermittent basis for ongoing maintenance of the vascular access device, drug and supply distribution, and assessment of clinical status and program compliance.

A major concern with the self-administration model is lack of medical supervision during the actual infusion. For example, anaphylaxis may occur with the initial dose of a drug. Anaphylactoid reactions may also occur with successive doses.[12] The patient or caregiver may inadvertently permit the medication to flow too rapidly, thereby causing fluid overload, electrolyte imbalance, or arrhythmias. The possibility of other drug reactions, such as the "red man syndrome" (flushing of the upper body) associated with vancomycin, is another reason for caution. For high-volume administration of some drugs— including vancomycin, amphotericin B, foscarnet, acyclovir, amino-glycosides, ganciclovir, and imipenem—a pump or rate-controlling device should be used. In this situation, patients are instructed to perform infusions only when a trained caregiver is present.

A second concern associated with self-administration or caregiver administration is sending patients home with an IV line in place. Although the potential for problems seems serious, they are actually unusual. However, patients should be selected carefully, trained well, and followed closely (see Chapter 2).

The extent to which the self-administration model is used will depend on the OPAT staff's expertise in patient training, available technology, and mandates for cost containment. The pressures of health care reform and capitation have resulted in the increasing popularity of this model. In some centers, self-administration has become the predominant method of delivering OPAT.

■ *The Home Infusion Company*

The most common method of OPAT delivery in the United States is actually a combination of the visiting nurse and self-administration models. Although this home-based OPAT is sometimes offered as an extension of an infusion center—whether hospital-based, hospital-affiliated, office-based, or offered by a visiting nurse service—it is more often coordinated by a commercial home infusion company, such as those that have proliferated throughout the United States.

Such companies, usually organized around pharmacy services, provide nurses and pharmacists with training and expertise in OPAT, medication, and IV equipment. Given their administrative structure, they can ensure quality drug delivery and utilize a system of third-party payment for medication with which insurance companies are familiar.

A hospital may contract with a home infusion company to assume all or part of the duties involved in delivering OPAT. The hospital may provide initial patient assessment and training, with the company carrying out the actual treatment at home. The hospital may provide nursing care as well, with the company responsible only for provision of pharmaceuticals and possibly expert infusion nurse backup and support. Finally, home infusion therapy also may be offered as one service of large home care agencies that deliver a variety of nursing services to home care patients.

Attending or referring physicians prescribe the drug to be given and for how long, as well as the clinical and laboratory parameters to be monitored throughout the course of treatment. Although each home infusion company has its own quality assurance guidelines, many have developed into large corporations in which physicians play only a peripheral role. The prescribing physician nevertheless bears ultimate responsibility for the care of the patient and outcome regardless of who administers the medication—nurse specialist, patient, or caregiver.[13,14] Thus, in prescribing OPAT, the doctor must ensure that patients enter quality programs, either provided in the physician's own office or through referral to an accredited hospital or independent agency known to be safe and effective.

■ *Health Maintenance Organizations*

The health maintenance organization (HMO) structure is well suited to the provision of OPAT. Patients can be referred from many sources, including primary care physicians, EDs, infectious disease consultants, nurses, pharmacists, and hospital discharge planners. Infusion services can be incorporated into existing operations, thus minimizing the need for additional staff. Reimbursement issues do not arise because all HMO services are automatically covered and physician supervision and control are usually ensured.[15]

■ *The OPAT Team*

Regardless of organizational structure, OPAT requires communication and coordination of effort between the prescribing physician, nurse specialist, pharmacist, and patient. Figure 1.2 describes the general responsibilities of each member of the team. Table 1.2 outlines the key elements required for an OPAT program.[3]

Physicians also may serve as medical directors of OPAT programs. A physician director can more easily than other medical professionals deal with the questions and problems of prescribing colleagues. Although the majority of home infusion companies are directed by pharmacists, physician directors are required by Medicare for any hospice home care program. The issue of physician certification or credentialing to provide OPAT is evolving. The American Academy of

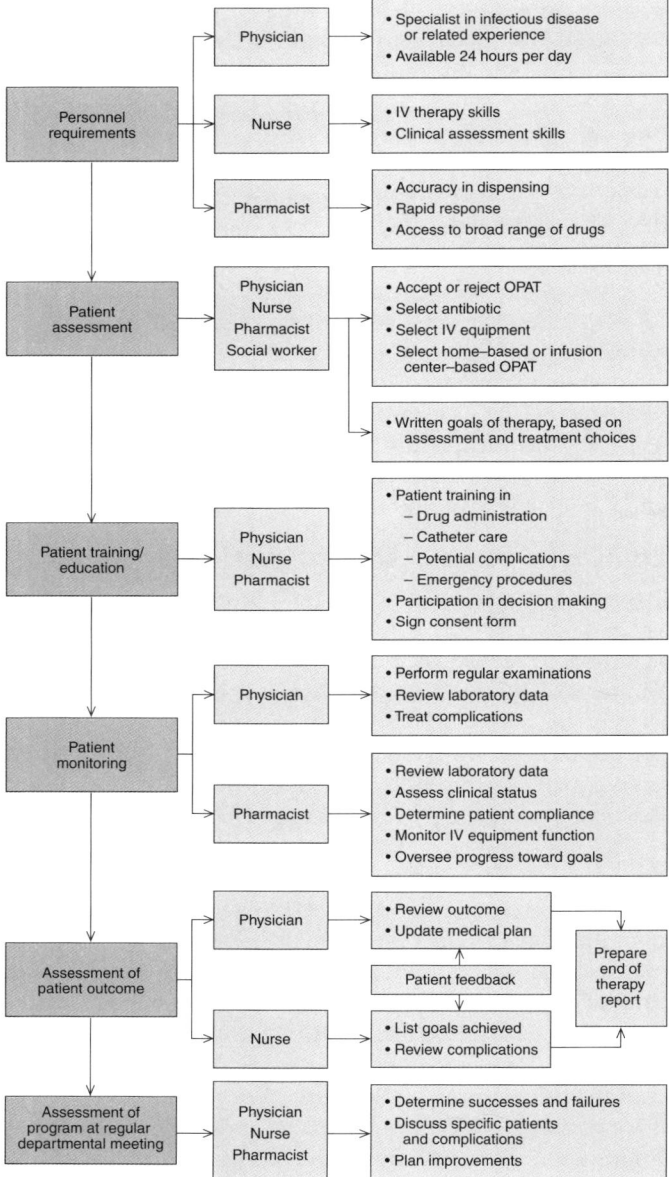

Figure 1.2. *The OPAT Team. (Adapted from Kunkel,* Hospital Practice, *Suppl. 1, 1993, with permission.)*

Table 1.2. Key Elements Required for an Outpatient Parenteral Antimicrobial Therapy (OPAT) Program

1. Health care team
   - A. An infectious diseases specialist or physician knowledgeable about infectious diseases and the use of antimicrobials in OPAT
   - B. Primary care or referring physicians available to participate in care
   - C. Nurse expert in IV therapy, access devices, and OPAT
   - D. Pharmacist knowledgeable about OPAT
   - E. Case manager and billing staff knowledgeable about therapeutic issues and third-party reimbursements
   - F. Access to other health care professionals, including a physical therapist, a dietitian, an occupational therapist, and a social worker

2. Communications
   - A. Physician, nurse, and pharmacist available 24 hours per day
   - B. System in place for rapid communication between patient and team members
   - C. Patient education information for common problems, side effects, precautions, and contact lists

3. Outline of guidelines for follow-up of patients with laboratory testing and intervention as needed

4. Written policies and procedures
   - A. Outline of responsibilities of team members
   - B. Patient intake information
   - C. Patient selection criteria
   - D. Patient education materials

5. Outcomes monitoring
   - A. Patient response
   - B. Complications of disease, treatment, or program
   - C. Patient satisfaction

Reprinted from Tice et al.,[3] with permission.

Home Care Physicians offers a certifying examination in home care.[16] Measurements of competence specific to the provision of OPAT are only a small part of a medical director's required credentials, however. For example, he or she should be knowledgeable and experienced in OPAT or certified by the American Board of Internal Medicine in infectious diseases, which requires the successful completion of an examination covering basic aspects and clinical features of infectious diseases, disease prevention and treatment, host defense mechanisms, and epidemiology.[17] Credentials in internal medicine and infectious diseases require training and education in outpatient care and patient management.

The Nurse

The infusion nurse specialist is responsible for[18-20]

- Inserting and maintaining vascular access devices
- Evaluating and recommending drug delivery devices
- Administering IV infusion
- Obtaining and evaluating laboratory samples
- Preventing and treating infusion-related complications
- Monitoring for compliance
- Monitoring for desired outcomes of therapy
- Promoting patient self-care through education
- Assisting patients with waste management
- Evaluating the home environment for safety
- Functioning as a patient advocate
- Keeping the physician informed of patient's progress

The nurse can contribute valuable input regarding drug dosing intervals and schedules, vascular access lines, and delivery systems based on the patient's venous status, lifestyle, mental and physical abilities, other clinical problems, and overall treatment plan.

Nurses may achieve specialty certification in infusion therapy through the Infusion Nurses Certification Corporation, the sister organization of the Infusion Nurses Society, which has established standards for nurses in all care settings.[18]

The Pharmacist

Pharmacists play a uniquely important role in the delivery of OPAT. Their responsibilities have been outlined by the American Society of Health-System Pharmacists (ASHP, formerly American Society of Hospital Pharmacists)[21-23] and often are regulated by state licensure laws as well as by standards set by the Joint Commission on Accreditation of Healthcare Organizations. The National Home Infusion Association offers certification in home infusion pharmacy. In most OPAT programs, pharmacist's responsibilities include the following:

- Assisting in the choice of drug and prescribed dosage
- Reviewing the patient's history of intolerant or allergic drug reactions
- Reviewing all other medications for interaction or toxicity

- Dispensing drugs and supplies
- Providing advice on drug stability and infusion-device technology
- Keeping staff and patients informed about potential adverse events
- Programming infusion pumps before delivery to patients as well as cleaning and maintaining the pumps
- Monitoring lab work and making recommendations regarding appropriate therapy

The ASHP has issued guidelines on the pharmacist's role in home care[21] and on the minimum standard for home care pharmacies,[22] both of which are available at http://www.ashp.org and in the 2005–2006 edition of the Society's publication *Best Practices for Hospital & Health-System Pharmacy. Position & Guidance Documents of ASHP.*[23]

The Patient and Caregiver

The patient and/or caregiver must be willing and able to comply with OPAT requirements. Those who do participate will be asked to assume a degree of responsibility that is vital to the quality, safety, and outcome of the treatment. Patients and caregivers are usually pleased to be involved in their own care and often come away with a sense of pride and satisfaction in their roles.

Other Team Members

Depending on the size, patient population, and organization of the OPAT program, other team members may include a social worker, an administrator or business manager, and a reimbursement specialist.[16,24]

A social worker can assess socioeconomic and insurance factors that may affect the effective delivery of OPAT and can arrange for ancillary support and services as needed.[25]

A laboratory technician and clinical microbiologist are needed to best perform appropriate studies and cultures for assessing the efficacy and potential toxicity of therapy. For example, patients taking β-lactam antibiotics should be monitored with complete blood counts at least once a week, and those receiving aminoglycosides or vancomycin should be followed with renal function tests twice a week.[16]

Expertise in reimbursement is central to success. The patient's insurance company should always be called for prior authorization to confirm that coverage is available and to determine the patient's copayment.

Finally, the third-party payer is for all intents and purposes another member of the OPAT team. The payer's regulations for coverage and reimbursement often determine how OPAT is provided or even if it is feasible. For example, Medicare will not always provide reimbursement for OPAT delivered in the home.

Once a patient has been evaluated, selected, and trained for OPAT, the work has just begun. The more difficult tasks are in following patients and ensuring the quality, safety, and outcome of treatment. In general, the standards for outpatient care are comparable to those for hospital care. Thus, a comprehensive plan for patient monitoring and follow-up is required for all OPAT programs.

References

1. Poretz DM. Outpatient parenteral antibiotic therapy. Management of serious infections. Part II: Amenable infections and models for delivery. Infusion center, office, and home. *Hosp Pract.* 1993;28(suppl 2):40–43.

2. Tice AD. Outpatient parenteral antibiotic therapy (OPAT) in the United States: delivery models and indications for use. *Can J Infect Dis.* 2000;11A:17A–21A.

3. Tice AD, Rehm SJ, Dalovisio JR, et al. Practice guidelines for outpatient parenteral antimicrobial therapy. IDSA guidelines. *Clin Infect Dis.* 2004;38:1651–1672.

4. Tice AD. Alternate site infusion: the physician-directed, office-based model. *J Intraven Nurs.* 1996;19:188–193.

5. Lindbeck G. Emergency department and urgent care center. *Hosp Pract.* 1993;28(suppl 2):44–47.

6. Nolet BR. Patient selection in outpatient parenteral antimicrobial therapy. *Infect Dis Clin North Am.* 1998;12:835–847.

7. Howard L, Michalek AV. Home parenteral nutrition (HPN). *Annu Rev Nutr.* 1984;4:69–99.

8. Ammann AJ, Ashman RF, Buckley RH, et al. Use of intravenous gamma-globulin in antibody immunodeficiency: results of a multicenter controlled trial. *Clin Immunol Immunopathol.* 1982;22:60–67.

9. Hayes N, Lovetang R. Home infusion therapy options for patients with AIDS. *Caring.* 1991;10:20–24.

10. Bradley JS, Ching DK, Phillips SE. Outpatient therapy of serious pediatric infections with ceftriaxone. *Pediatr Infect Dis J.* 1988;7:160–164.

11. Stiver HG, Trosky SK, Cote DD, et al. Self-administration of IV antibiotics: an efficient cost-effective home care program. *Can Med Assoc J.* 1996;127:107–111.

12. Kunkel MJ, Tice AD, OPIVITA Study Group. Serious adverse events in outpatient parenteral antibiotic therapy: a prospective multicenter study [abstract]. *Proc Infect Dis Soc Am.* 1995;132:1.

13. *Wickline v State of California*, Court of Appeal 2nd Dist, Div 5 (July 30, 1986). 192 Cal App 3rd 1630. 239 Cal. Rptr. 810.

14. National Intravenous Therapy Association's Intravenous Nursing Standards of Practice. *NITA.* 1984;7:93.

15. Eron LJ. Parenteral antibiotic therapy in outpatients: quality assurance and other issues in a protohospital. *Chemotherapy.* 1991;37(suppl 2):14–20.

16. American Academy of Health Care Physicians. Home care credentialing examination. AAHCP Website. Available at: www.aahcp.org. Accessed October 8, 2004.

17. American Board of Internal Medicine. Infectious disease exam. Requirements for certification. ABIM Website. Available at: www.abim.org/cert/ssid.shtm. Accessed May 31, 2005.

18. Infusion Nurses Society. Infusion nursing standards of practice. *J Intraven Nurs.* 2000;23(suppl 6):S1– S88.

19. Lonsway RA. Intravenous therapy in the home. In: Hankins J, Lonsway RA, Hedrick C, Perdue M, eds. *Infusion Therapy in Clinical Practice.* 2nd ed. Philadelphia, Pa: WB Saunders; 2001:501–534.

20. Mortlock N. Intravenous therapy in the alternative care setting. Ibid:535–560.

21. American Society of Health-System Pharmacists. ASHP guidelines on the pharmacist's role in home care. *Am J Health Syst Pharm.* 2000;57:1252–1257.

22. McKinnon B, Bertch KE, Carey LP, et al. ASHP guidelines: minimum standard for home care pharmacies. American Society of Health-System Pharmacists. *Am J Health Syst Pharm.* 1999;56:629–638.

23. American Society of Health-System Pharmacists. *Best Practices for Hospital & Health-System Pharmacy. Position & Guidance Documents of ASHP.* 2005–2006 ed. Bethesda, MD: American Society of Health-System Pharmacists.

24. Rehm SJ, Weinstein AJ. Home intravenous antibiotic therapy: a team approach. *Ann Intern Med.* 1983;99:388–392.

25. Sharp JW. Social work in a home intravenous antibiotic therapy program. *Soc Work Health Care.* 1986;12:93–101.

CHAPTER 2

Patient Selection and Education

Although no hard-and-fast rules govern the selection of patients for outpatient parenteral antimicrobial therapy (OPAT), several essential, interrelated criteria are generally taken into account (Figure 2.1).[1] Clinical factors are, of course, the most important (Table 2.1).[2] The list of clinical conditions that can be treated outside the hospital lengthens as sicker patients with more severe infections are assigned or discharged to outpatient care and newer, more potent antibiotics become available. See Chapter 3 for a detailed discussion of infections usually treated with OPAT and Chapter 4 for the pharmacodynamics and pharmacokinetics of the relevant pharmaceutical agents.

Most infections can be treated, at least in part, outside the hospital. Patients with possible sepsis, endocarditis, meningitis, or septic arthritis should be hospitalized until the infection is under control. Even then, their overall condition may be medically inappropriate for OPAT because of concomitant diseases, such as diabetes, renal failure, heart disease, or drug addiction. Outpatient care also may be impossible for patients who require additional nursing care, particularly those with orthopedic disabilities, severe pain, incontinence, or dementia.

Initiation of OPAT requires that the consulting or primary physician determines that such therapy is needed to treat a defined infection, that hospitalization is not needed to control the infection, and that alternate routes of drug delivery are not feasible or appropriate.[2]

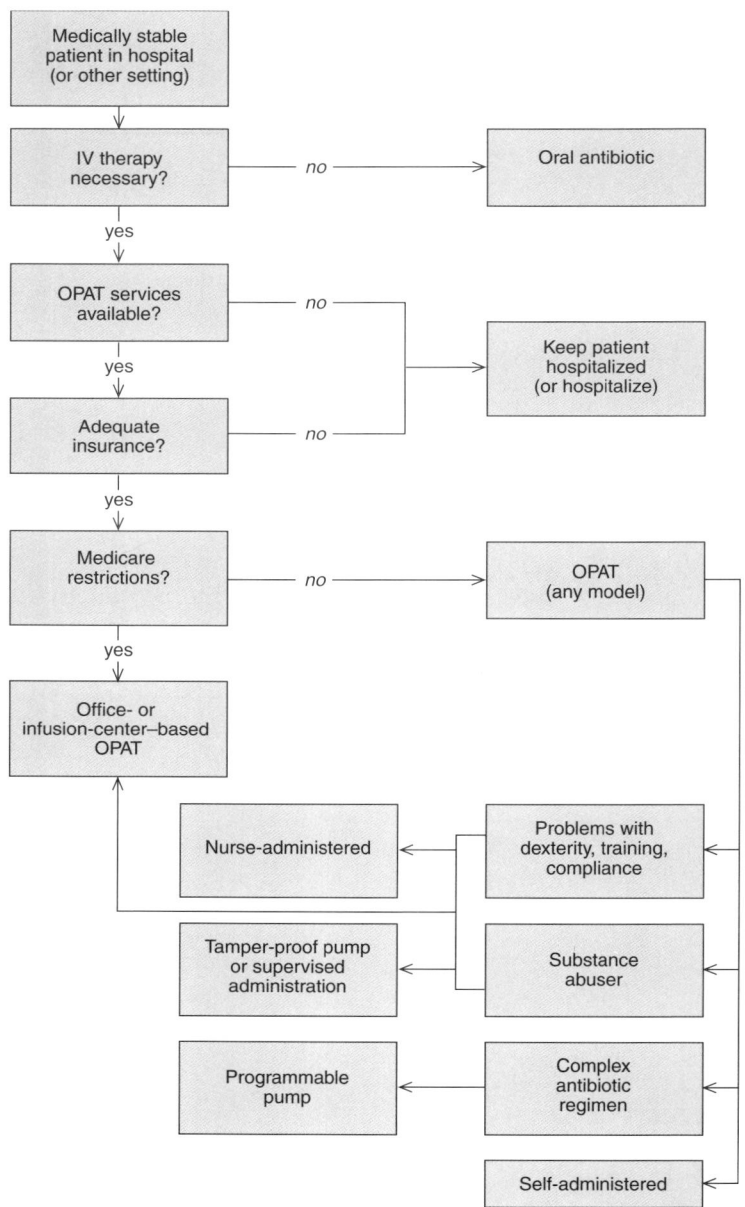

Figure 2.1. Patient Selection for OPAT.
(From Brown,[1] with permission.)

Table 2.1. Specific Considerations in Evaluating Patients for Outpatient Parenteral Antimicrobial Therapy (OPAT)

1. Is parenteral antimicrobial therapy needed?
2. Do the patient's medical care needs exceed resources available at the proposed site of care?
3. Is the home or outpatient environment safe and adequate to support care?
4. Are the patient and/or caregiver willing to participate and able to safely, effectively, and reliably deliver parenteral antimicrobial therapy?
5. Are mechanisms for rapid and reliable communications about problems and for monitoring of therapy in place among members of the OPAT team?
6. Do the patient and caregiver understand the benefits, risks, and economic considerations involved in OPAT?
7. Does informed consent need to be documented?

Reprinted from Tice et al.,[3] with permission.

■ *Patient/Caregiver Attitudes*

Once the physician decides that a patient's infection and condition are appropriate for OPAT, he or she must consider the patient's and caregiver's desires and attitudes. Is the idea of administering intravenous (IV) therapy outside the hospital acceptable? Is it frightening? Does a hospitalized patient feel he or she is being discharged simply for monetary reasons? Such concerns must be addressed because the success of OPAT is fundamentally dependent on the patient's and caregiver's willingness to participate, ability to understand its inherent complications and potential problems, and ability to learn the necessary skills.

Mental and Physical Abilities

The mental abilities of a patient or caregiver, particularly as related to the level of self-confidence, anxiety, and fears, should be assessed by the attending or prescribing physician. The OPAT delivery team may also wish to conduct an informal psychosocial evaluation of the patient's or caregiver's mental status. It should be noted that a stable, nondebilitating psychiatric illness need not interfere with OPAT delivery and should not preclude his or her participation.

Physical abilities are another consideration. Limitations in walking, prolonged sitting, and access to transportation may weigh against outpatient treatment. Even the visiting nurse model may not be appropriate for patients who live alone and are unable to bathe themselves or take care of other basic activities of daily living; however, for such patients, some third-party payers may include personal care assistance by unlicensed personnel.

The risk of IV narcotic or other drug abuse must always be considered in patient selection. Drug abusers may use an IV line for drugs not prescribed, but prolonged hospitalization may be difficult to justify and may not necessarily prevent the problem. Therefore, any suspicion of potential drug abuse should be tempered by the prescribing physician's judgment of the patient's ability to comply with the treatment plan. In case of doubts, abuse-proof delivery models should be considered (see Chapter 6).

■ Reimbursement Issues

Patients and families should be counseled about reimbursement issues, particularly if the patient will be required to pay some of the cost. For example, some health insurance companies insist that patients be discharged if hospitalization is not essential, yet they do not cover outpatient costs. Other payers may pay for 100% of hospital charges but only 80% of outpatient costs, despite the fact that OPAT is much less costly than an extended hospital stay. In either case, patients may prefer to stay in the hospital for continuing IV therapy.

Financial resources to support other aspects of treatment also must be addressed. Outpatient parenteral care may not be a viable option for patients who are not able financially to maintain basic nutrition, other medications, or wound care supplies.

■ The Home Situation

One of the most important aspects of a home situation is the availability of family support. This makes a program much safer and more effective. Although patients who live alone can also be considered for OPAT, they should be encouraged to stay with a responsible friend or relative during treatment.

The social situation at home is also an important component of successful OPAT. In the presence of marital problems or already demanding responsibilities for the care of children or elderly parents, patients may be better off remaining hospitalized for the parenteral phase of antimicrobial therapy.

It is crucial to gain at least some knowledge of the patient's home environment through inspection or inquiry. The self-administration model requires that patients have running water for hand washing. A telephone line or cellular phone is considered essential for ready communication with the prescribing physician and the OPAT provider. For self-administered OPAT, a refrigerator is usually necessary for storage of prepared antimicrobials.

Ready access to transportation is also important. Patients should have an automobile and the ability to drive or should have ready access to a car and driver or other transportation. Patients at risk for acute medical emergencies, such as those with endocarditis who live an hour or more from medical care, should not be considered for outpatient therapy.

■ *Patient Education*

As essential members of the OPAT team, patients and their caregivers must be well-informed and willing participants. They must understand the risks and responsibilities associated with outpatient therapy. They should know, for example, that they assume potentially life-threatening risks in leaving the hospital. They must be informed about the infection, its treatment, and the potential problems to look for. Written materials about OPAT—ideally, in simple language with pictures or graphics—should be provided for later review and reference. Some commercially available patient education materials can be adapted for teaching the required skills. The fundamentals of a patient education curriculum are listed in Table 2.2.[3]

Preparing patients or caregivers to assume responsibility for independent IV administration is a major part of the role of the OPAT team's infusion nurse specialist.[3,4] Medicare regulations consider patient teaching "skilled nursing" if the material requires the skills and knowledge of a professional, is necessary, and leads to patient independence.[5]

The nurse can begin teaching during actual administration of an infusion, thus enabling evaluation of the patient's or caregiver's willingness and ability to learn, as well as his or her understanding of the diagnosis and acceptance of the treatment regimen while monitoring

Table 2.2.   Topics for Patient Education in OPAT

• Purpose of therapy	• Therapeutic monitoring procedures
• Infection control	• Supply management
• Solutions, medications, and formulas	• Complications
• Administration procedures	• Emergency interventions
• Vascular access care	• Special instructions

From Baranowski and Pierce,[3] with permission.

the patient's response to medication. Early identification of a patient's or caregiver's fears or aversions—to needles or blood, for example—may be crucial to the success of the home care program. This is also the time for the nurse to look for physical impediments to independence, including impaired visual acuity, manual dexterity, or limited mobility. The determination of an able, willing, and dependable caregiver may be the nurse's most difficult and most crucial assessment.

Patients may be introduced to home infusion therapy in a variety of alternative settings—the physician's office, an infusion center, a hospital emergency department, or even at home. Teaching plans need to be individualized according to type of therapy, venous access, drug delivery system, and home environment. Presentation should include discussion and demonstration of aspects of therapy, including possible adverse effects, such as bleeding and phlebitis. Illustrations are particularly helpful, as are materials that permit patients to handle the equipment and practice technique with models. Most patients and caregivers can be taught to administer infusions in a single 2-hour session. Telemedicine with home monitors or interactive audio/video devices for home assessment and compliance may be helpful.[6]

Sterile technique and any problems that patients or caregivers have had with IV line maintenance or flushing procedures should be reviewed during every nursing visit or scheduled appointment. Infection control is also an important area of education, especially with regard to draining wounds and disposal of infected material and needles.[7,8]

■ *Access to Medical Staff*

A safe and effective OPAT program must have a physician, nurse, and pharmacist on call 24 hours a day, 7 days a week. Patients should have clear, written instructions as to whom and what numbers to call with what problems and under what circumstances.

References

1. Brown RB. Selecting the patient. *Hosp Pract.* 1993;28(suppl 1):11–15.

2. Tice AD, Rehm SJ. Dalovisio JR, et al. Practice guidelines for outpatient parenteral antimicrobial therapy. IDSA guidelines. *Clin Infect Dis.* 2004;38:1651–1672.

3. Baranowski L, Pierce CA. The role of the home infusion nurse. In: Conners RB, Winters RW, eds. *Home Infusion: Current Status and Future Trends.* Chicago, IL: Health Forum; 1995:19–34.

4. Tice AD. Alternate site infusion: the physician-directed, office-based model. *J Intraven Nurs.* 1996;19:188–193.

5. Health Care Financing Administration. *Medicare Home Health Agency Manual.* HCFA Publication 11. Washington, DC: U.S. Government Printing Office, 2004. Available at: www.cms.hhs.gov/manuals/11_hha/hh100.asp. Accessed May 18, 2005.

6. Eron LJ, Marineau M, Baclig E, et al. The virtual hospital: treating acute infections in the home by telemedicine. *Hawaii Med J.* 2004;63:291–293.

7. Bower J, Segarra-Newnham M, Tice A. Selecting change implementation strategies. In: Mayhall CG, ed. *Hospital Epidemiology and Infection Control.* 3rd ed. Philadelphia, Pa: Lippincott Williams & Wilkins; 2004;161–174.

8. Tice AD, Barrett T. Home health care. In: Abrutyn E, Goldmann DA, Sheckler WE, eds. *Saunders Infection Control Reference Service. The Experts' Guide to the Guidelines.* 2nd ed. Philadelphia, Pa: WB Saunders; 2001:151–197.

CHAPTER 3

Infections Amenable to Outpatient Parenteral Antimicrobial Therapy

Decisions regarding which infections are appropriate to treat on an outpatient basis vary with the institution, the prescribing physician, and the individual patient's condition and wishes. Infections that are commonly treated with outpatient parenteral antimicrobial therapy (OPAT) are discussed here, with emphasis on how therapy may differ from that in the inpatient setting.

■ Endocarditis

An estimated 5000 to 8000 new cases of endocarditis are diagnosed in the United States each year, approximately half of which are caused by penicillin-susceptible streptococci.[1] Staphylococci also play a significant causative role, and a number of other organisms, including the HACEK species (*Haemophilus*, *Actinobacillus*, *Cardiobacterium*, *Eikenella*, and *Kingella*), are involved to a much lesser degree.

Endocarditis primarily affects people with preexisting heart disease, such as mitral valve prolapse, those with prosthetic heart valves, and those who are intravenous (IV) drug abusers. Because the infection is associated with a high rate of morbidity and mortality, hospitalization was once considered mandatory. With the availability of safer, more effective infusion devices and improved antimicrobial agents with prolonged half-lives, outpatient therapy has become possible, even preferable, in many cases.

Many patients with streptococcal endocarditis, including some with enterococcal disease, are candidates for OPAT.[2-4] Those with more aggressive staphylococcal disease are at greater risk for complications, but some can be discharged to OPAT after initial evaluation and stabilization in the hospital. Intravenous drug abusers with right-sided endocarditis have a better prognosis than those with left-sided involvement. They may be discharged earlier if cardiac studies fail to show an abscess or conduction abnormality.

Patients infected with gram-negative bacteria or multiple organisms are at greater risk with OPAT because their course is not as predictable. Patients with any of the HACEK group organisms often may be treated at home, because these organisms are usually very sensitive to antibiotics. The only caveat about these patients is that they may have a higher potential for embolization. It has been suggested that patients with uncomplicated endocarditis due to viridans group streptococci could be discharged to receive OPAT after 1 week of hospitalization.[4]

Treatment Regimen

The traditional course of treatment for endocarditis is 4 to 6 weeks of IV antibiotic(s) to which the causative organism is susceptible. Most viridans streptococci and nonenterococcal group D streptococci, such as *Streptococcus bovis*, are sensitive to penicillin and may be treated for only 2 weeks with a β-lactam and an aminoglycoside antibiotic.[5] For the stable patient at low risk for complications, most or all of the antibiotic course can be administered as OPAT.

Before a patient with endocarditis is sent home from the hospital, a number of potential problems should be considered, including the development of systemic emboli, valve failure, or cardiac rhythm disturbances. In patients with rhythm disturbances, infection of the conduction system should be suspected, and they should remain hospitalized with a cardiac monitor and staff readily available to deal with any life-threatening arrhythmia. The possibility of heart failure must also be considered, particularly if the infection destroys a valve or its supporting structures. Because emergency surgical intervention may be necessary in this situation, patients should have ready access to emergency services and a hospital with cardiac surgery facilities.

Emboli to the brain or essential organs are not uncommon in left-sided infections, particularly in the presence of large vegetations or of certain organisms, such as *Haemophilus aphrophilus*.

The risks associated with causative organisms should also be considered before patients are sent home. Streptococci are less likely to cause myocardial abscesses and destroy valves than the more aggressive *Staphylococcus aureus*, which may burrow into the myocardium to create fistulas as well as dysrhythmias.

Because of such potential complications, discharge to OPAT may not be wise unless patients have a companion or caregiver and live within a short distance of emergency medical care.

Reliable vascular access is a particularly important factor in endocarditis therapy because interruptions in treatment should be avoided. Central lines are often placed to accommodate long-term therapy as well as to avoid phlebitis caused by drugs such as vancomycin, oxacillin, and penicillin. Long lines should not be placed, however, until the bacteria have been cleared.

■ Osteomyelitis

Infections of the bone lend themselves well to OPAT because patients are often otherwise healthy, and a prolonged 4- to 6-week course of treatment is necessary.[6,7] Studies of OPAT conducted at Infections Limited indicate that the likelihood of failure and amputation are higher with concomitant diabetes and vascular disease but not clearly with the factor of age.[8] The length of treatment depends on the extent and depth of the infection, the bones and organisms involved, host factors, and the patient's age. Uncomplicated osteomyelitis in children, for example, responds well to 1 or 2 weeks of IV antimicrobial therapy followed by oral agents (if adequate serum levels can be reached) for another 2 to 4 weeks.[9] It is useful to obtain serum bactericidal levels on oral as well as parenteral antimicrobials to be certain their activity is adequate and to adjust the dose if necessary.

Diskitis with vertebral osteomyelitis in the adult, on the other hand, is a deep, serious, and difficult-to-treat infection that does not lend itself well to surgical intervention. Standard recommendations are IV infusion of antimicrobial agents for a minimum of 6 weeks. Patients may also experience such severe pain and spasm that they are kept in the hospital for pain control and subsequent physical therapy. They are often in a cumbersome body jacket or cast as well, to limit the motion of the spine. For those who are treated as outpatients, the visiting nurse or self-administration model may be the best-choice setting because of the pain associated with getting out of bed to go to an infusion center.

Hospitalization should be considered for osteomyelitis patients with complicating diseases, such as diabetes, neuropathy, arterial insufficiency, and recent trauma, or when there are concerns about self-care.

Infecting Organisms

Although the primary bacterial cause of osteomyelitis is *S. aureus*, coagulase-negative staphylococci may be involved in foreign body infections, such as those around a prosthetic joint. Gram-negative osteomyelitis may occur as a result of hematogenous spread from injuries and surgical wounds, IV drug abuse, and, occasionally, sepsis or urinary infections. Information from the OPAT Outcomes Registry indicates that the most common bacteria causing osteomyelitis are methicillin-sensitive *S. aureus* (78%), methicillin-resistant *S. aureus* (16%), coagulase-negative staphylococci (15%), and gram-negative rods (14%).[7]

Methicillin-resistant staphylococci (either coagulase-positive or coagulase-negative) have become an increasing challenge with vancomycin, currently the only available agent for treating osteomyelitis. Recently, however, several new antistaphylococcal antibiotics have become available, although not yet approved for treatment of osteomyelitis by the Food and Drug Administration. Daptomycin is a new parenteral agent that can be given once daily. Linezolid can be given by mouth as well as intravenously but is not as bactericidal as vancomycin. Many more expensive and lengthy clinical trials and cooperative efforts will be needed to determine the optimal antimicrobial regimen for the treatment of osteomyelitis.

Antibiotic Therapy

Although most gram-negative bone infections can be treated with an oral quinolone,[10] some strains of *Pseudomonas* and *Enterobacter* have become resistant to quinolone and thus require traditional parenteral therapy (Figure 3.1). Furthermore, oral quinolones are not appropriate for children because of the drugs' potentially adverse effects on growing joints.[9] Failures with OPAT have also been higher with *Pseudomonas aeruginosa* than with staphylococci or streptococci.[7]

The efficacy of antibiotic therapy in osteomyelitis correlates well with drug Schlichter test levels (serum bactericidal concentrations) of 1:2 or greater at the trough in adults, 1:8 or greater in children.[9] Thus, sustained drug levels carry a theoretical benefit, as do antibiotic agents with longer half-lives, such as some of the cephalosporins.

Continuous infusion or multiple dosing of drugs with short half-lives (e.g., oxacillin or nafcillin) via a pump and central venous line may be equally effective but less adaptable to home therapy. Combined therapy is also possible with, for example, both a β-lactam or

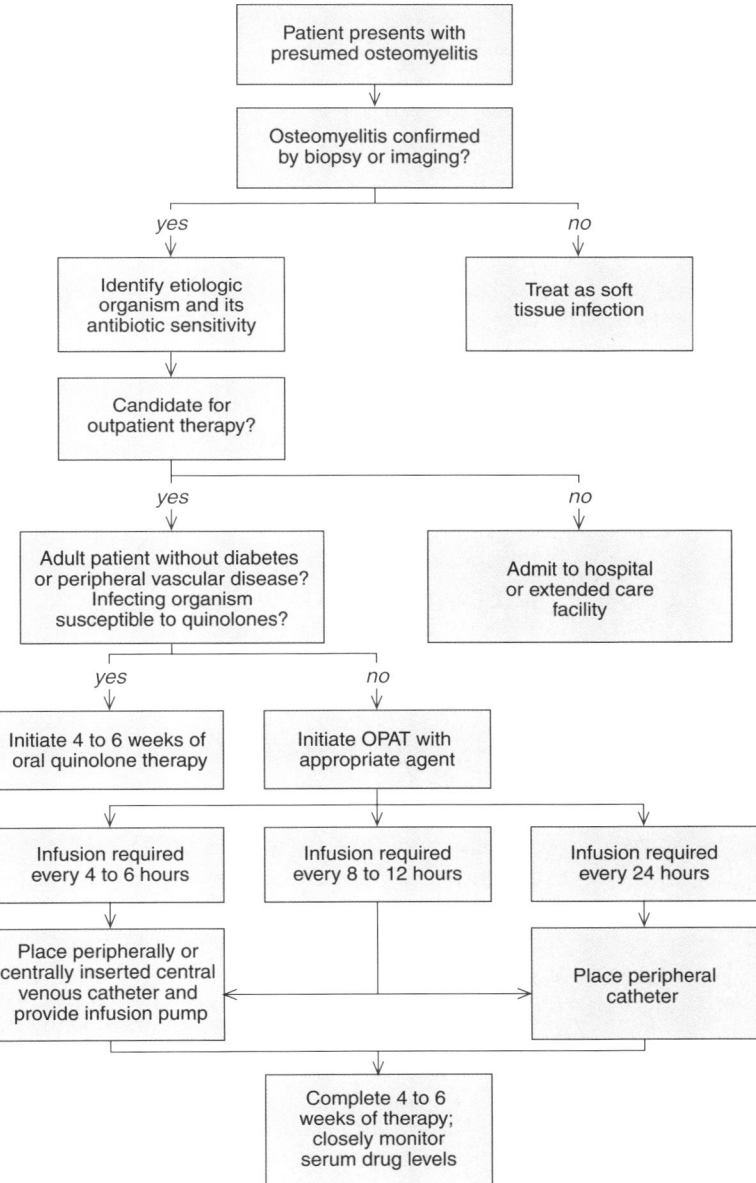

Figure 3.1. *Outpatient Therapy for Osteomyelitis. (From Tice,[6] with permission.)*

a carbapenems and an aminoglycoside agent for Pseudomonas or resistant *Enterobacter* infections.

Infections associated with surgery, such as infection of a tibial fracture that has been plated, should be treated like osteomyelitis. Initial considerations might include immediate removal of the plate with placement of an external stabilization device. As a rule, however, the hardware is left in place until the infection is brought under control. In many cases, the infection can be treated or suppressed until bone healing and union is sufficient to permit its removal. In either case, a prolonged course of IV antimicrobial therapy is often needed in such patients, who may otherwise be well, healthy, and anxious to leave the hospital.

Surgery

Surgical intervention may be necessary when there is dead tissue or devitalized bone or if the infection involves the soft tissue and is progressing rapidly. Removal of dead tissue not only allows for faster healing but may prevent the development of resistant organisms. In fact, quinolone resistance may develop during active treatment of gram-negative osteomyelitis if the focus of infection is not removed. Surgery should also be considered to correct or restore vascular supply when perfusion is poor.

■ Wound Infections

Infections may complicate a variety of wounds, from soft tissue trauma to surgery. Depending on the depth of injury and the tissues involved, IV antimicrobial therapy may be necessary. Wounds caused by heavy blows or bullets, which often involve significant tissue damage, provide fertile ground for a wide variety of infecting organisms. Such infections may require debridement as well as prolonged aggressive parenteral therapy with high concentrations of antimicrobials. Bite wounds, particularly of the hand, or wounds caused by fist-to-mouth injuries are also prone to severe infections requiring IV antimicrobials and early surgery.

Infecting Organisms

The organisms involved in wound infections vary considerably. Community-acquired infections are often caused by *S. aureus*, streptococci and, at times, anaerobes, depending on the site and type of injury. Surgical wound infections present a greater challenge, given the presence of resistant organisms bred in the hospital and selected by perioperative antimicrobial therapy. Such bacteria may vary from the gram-negative, such as *Enterobacter, Pseudomonas, Acinetobacter* species, and *Escherichia coli*, to the resistant gram-positive, including methicillin-resistant *S. aureus*, coagulase-negative staphylococci, and enterococci, some of which are resistant to vancomycin.

Regardless of how and where acquired, wound infections should be cultured, although surface swabs may not reflect the real, deeper pathogens. Treatment will depend on the identification and antimicrobial sensitivity of the recovered organisms. For example, an infected bite wound often involves a spectrum of organisms, from streptococci to facultative and strict anaerobes. Although several antimicrobial regimens would provide good coverage, agents permitting less frequent dosing are obviously more appropriate for outpatient treatment.

Ampicillin/sulbactam provides a broad spectrum of coverage for infections due to bites, but the combination is not very stable once it is mixed and so must be prepared daily, thus complicating home treatment. A combination of ceftriaxone with clindamycin also will provide good coverage for a bite-wound infection, but clindamycin should be administered every 8 hours. Finally, metronidazole, which is very active against most anaerobic organisms and is absorbed very well by mouth, can be substituted for clindamycin in the ceftriaxone combination. Metronidazole has a half-life of approximately 10 hours, even longer than that of ceftriaxone and, thus, needs to be given only once or twice a day. Ertapenem can provide a full spectrum of anaerobic and aerobic activity in a single daily dose.[11]

For infections acquired in the hospital, empiric therapy should include vancomycin or daptomycin to cover methicillin-resistant staphylococci and enterococci. If a Gram stain shows gram-negative organisms, a third-generation cephalosporin, such as ceftazidime, should be considered, particularly if *Pseudomonas* sp. is a concern.

■ *Skin, Skin Structure, and Soft Tissue Infections*

In the past, standard practice has been to hospitalize patients with serious soft tissue infections, such as cellulitis, lymphangitis, and abscesses. Then, after being stabilized, the patients are discharged with prescriptions for continuing treatment with oral antimicrobials. With the introduction and development of OPAT, these patients are being considered for outpatient care much earlier, often without hospital admission.[12-14] Hospital emergency rooms increasingly initiate IV antimicrobial therapy and either refer patients to established OPAT programs or develop their own centers.[15]

Infecting Organisms

Most skin and soft tissue infections are caused by streptococci or staphylococci. Until recently, the community-acquired staphylococci were susceptible to once-daily antibiotics such as ceftriaxone and ertapenem. However, with the growing resistance of S. aureus in the community to methicillin and even vancomycin, newer parenteral drugs, such as daptomycin and linezolid, must be considered.[16] An oral quinolone can be used as well if gram-negative coverage is also necessary. Oral metronidazole can be added if anaerobic organisms are suspected.

■ HIV-Associated Infections

Secondary or opportunistic infections present a serious challenge to patients infected with HIV. Chronic and recurrent infections, such as cytomegalovirus retinitis, Toxoplasma encephalitis, and deep fungal infections with Candida, Histoplasma, and Coccidioides often require prolonged courses of IV therapy. With the advent of effective antiretroviral therapy, these infections have come under control, and the immune system that prevents their occurrence has often been restored.

For patients who remain immunosuppressed and, therefore, need initial or prolonged IV therapy, home and outpatient therapy is an obvious need.[17] Some AIDS patients refuse hospitalization altogether and will take virtually any risk to stay at home with friends and family. Thus, the medical system is being asked to provide in an outpatient setting potentially toxic medications that require close medical supervision. The situation is complicated by the progressive nature of HIV-associated infections, the currently limited expectations for a cure, and, as the immune system wanes, the development of infections that are increasingly refractory to therapy.

Many fungal infections should be treated initially with amphotericin B. However, once a response to the drug has been achieved, oral agents such as fluconazole, voraconazole, and itraconazole may be as effective. Acyclovir, ganciclovir, foscarnet, and cidofovir may be needed for cytomegalovirus[18] or herpes.[19] A new parenteral antiviral, enfuvirtide (T-20), has recently become available for advanced HIV infection and can be given once daily also.[20]

Cytomegalovirus

Cytomegalovirus is a major challenge, with ganciclovir, cidofovir, and foscarnet the main regimens of therapy found to be effective. Intravenous ganciclovir has played a major role in HIV care, but with better oral agents, such as valganciclovir[21] and highly active antiretroviral therapy, its use has fallen dramatically. For an acute infection, however, a 2- or 3-week induction course of ganciclovir with infusions of the drug twice a day may be indicated. If ganciclovir resistance develops, patients may be switched to foscarnet or cidofovir for another induction phase followed by lifetime maintenance.

Treatment of HIV-related infections has been greatly facilitated by a variety of reliable vascular access devices, particularly peripherally inserted central catheters (PICCs).[22] In some patients, a single PICC has been used for ganciclovir infusions for a year or more.

In general, there is good community support for the home treatment of AIDS patients. Patients often are capable of self-administration of drugs and, as their condition deteriorates, many are helped by family, friends, and volunteers from community organizations. As the patient population shifts to a higher percentage of IV drug users, children, prisoners, and others with few socioeconomic resources, careful patient selection will become crucial for the continued success of OPAT.

◼ *Lower Respiratory Tract Infections*

The first report of outpatient IV antimicrobial therapy, by Rucker and Harrison in 1974, involved lower respiratory tract infections in children with cystic fibrosis (CF).[23] Since then, OPAT has become standard therapy for both children and adults with CF. Comparison of OPAT with inpatient treatment of these patients shows outpatient treatment to be preferable on three major counts: reduced cost, improved quality of life, and less risk of cross-contamination with resistant organisms.

◼ *Community-Acquired Pneumonia*

An empiric parenteral antibiotic for patients with pneumonia serious enough to be hospitalized is standard. Both the Infectious Diseases Society of America and the American Thoracic Society have advocated the use of ceftriaxone for empiric therapy.[24,25] This advice has been taken one step further by Medicare as a quality assurance measure that advocates an infusion within 4 hours of evaluation in an emergency room for patients who are admitted.[26,27]

Decisions about admission to a hospital and hence the route of administration were evaluated in a study of more than 14,000 patients, from which the investigators derived a prediction rule, the Pneumonia Severity Index (PSI), which stratified patients into five classes with respect to the risk of death within 30 days.[28] The higher the score, the higher the risk of death, admission to the intensive care unit, and readmission and, consequently, the longer the stay (Figure 3.2).[29] The decision regarding initial site of treatment can be made using a systematic two-step process.[29,30]

Step one involves assessment of any preexisting conditions that compromise the safety of home care, including severe hemodynamic instability, active coexisting conditions that require hospitalization, acute hypoxemia or chronic oxygen dependency, and inability to take oral medications. The second step involves calculation of the PSI, with patients in risk classes I, II, or III recommended for home care. Although the use of oral antibiotics while hospitalized and parenteral antibiotics as outpatients were not assessed, the classifications system provided useful information in evaluating patients with pneumonia for OPAT. The duration of therapy for pneumonia and the need for combined therapy with a macrolide or simply a quinolone alone remains debatable. Decisions about OPAT must remain with the individual patient and the resources available.[31-33]

When to switch from IV to oral antibiotic therapy for pneumonia is also under evaluation. This is an important economic factor, as OPAT is not always available for early hospital discharge and is more expensive than most oral drugs. Ramirez[34] and others have demonstrated the safety of early switch from IV therapy to oral antibiotics, but the timing and total duration of therapy need further study.

■ *Other Infections*

Virtually every infection can be treated with OPAT for at least part of a course of IV therapy. Intravenous antimicrobials also may be useful for providing prophylaxis before dental work in patients with prosthetic heart valves.

With continued use and experience, OPAT will undoubtedly be used to treat increasingly severe infections effectively and safely. For example, in a recent study, 200 patients with cellulitis who had no contraindications for home care were assigned to receive treatment either at home or in hospital.[35] Days to no advancement of cellulitis was the primary outcome measure, with days on IV and oral antibiotics, days in hospital or home care, complications, degree of functioning and pain, and satisfac-

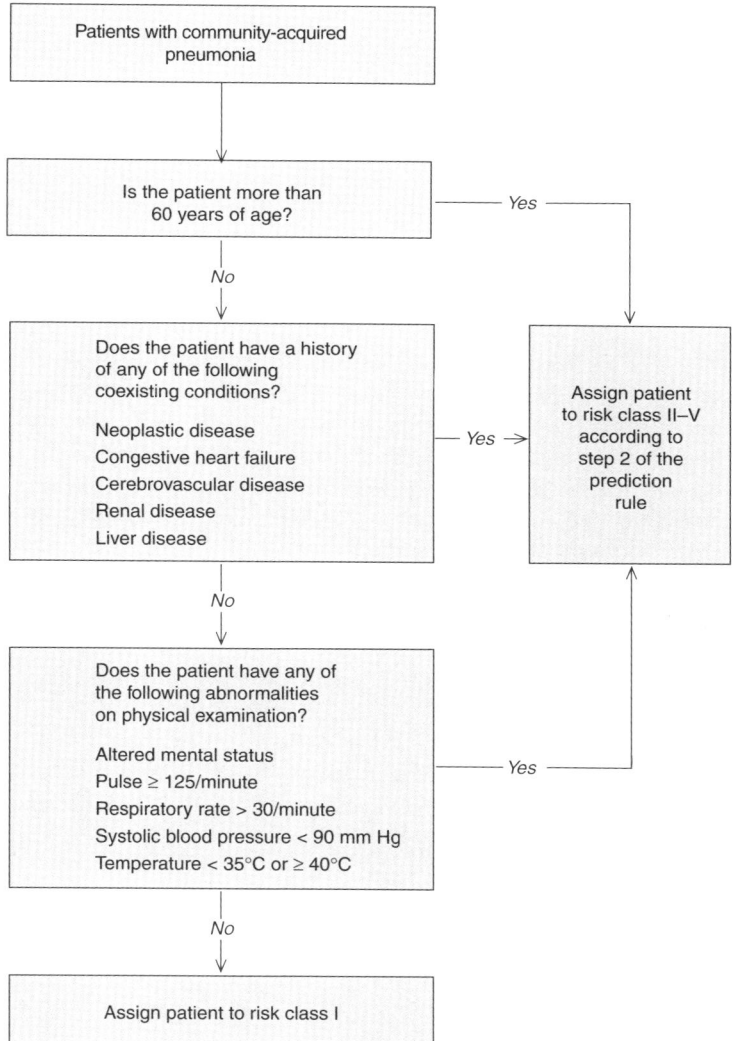

Figure 3.2. *The Pneumonia Severity Index. (From Halm and Teirstein,[29] with permission.)*

tion with site of care also recorded. The two treatment groups did not differ significantly for the primary or any other outcome measure except for patient satisfaction, which was greater in those treated at home.

Another trial followed 100 patients treated with 107 courses of OPAT for bone and joint infections, diskitis/osteomyelitis, septic arthritis, and metalware/prosthetic joint infections.[36] All but 6 patients self-administered up to 4 times daily. The majority of complications were minor, and 88% of patients were cured.

Meningitis

All meningitis patients should be hospitalized initially, but once clinically stabilized, they can usually complete the 10- to 14-day course of antimicrobial therapy as outpatients.

Urinary Tract Infections

Urinary tract infections with organisms resistant to oral medications may respond well to once-a-day IV or intramuscular injections of aminoglycosides or cephalosporins. Pyelonephritis caused by the usual organisms, such as *E. coli,* may respond more rapidly to IV than oral agents and may be easily treated with single daily doses of ceftriaxone, gentamicin, or tobramycin.[37]

Abdominal/Pelvic Abscesses

Abdominal and pelvic abscesses may be treated, at least in part, in an outpatient setting, although surgery may often be necessary. For some abscesses, a week's course of IV antimicrobial therapy may be well tolerated and make surgery far easier and safer than initial exploration of the phlegmon. Pelvic inflammatory disease often responds well to OPAT. Even tubo-ovarian abscesses have been known to resolve without surgical intervention.[38]

References

1. Wilson WR, Karchmer AW, Dajani AS, et al. Antibiotic treatment of adults with infective endocarditis due to streptococci, enterococci, staphylococci, and HACEK microorganisms. *JAMA.* 1995;274:1706–1713.

2. Rehm SJ. Outpatient intravenous antibiotic therapy for endocarditis. *Infect Dis Clin North Am.* 1998;12:879–901.

3. Karchmer AW. Outpatient management of infective endocarditis. *Infect Med.* 1994;11(suppl C):8–11.

4. Andrews MM, von Reyn CF. Patient selection criteria and management guidelines for outpatient parenteral antibiotic therapy for native valve infective endocarditis. *Clin Infect Dis.* 2001;33:203–209.

5. Sexton DJ, Tenenbaum MJ, Wilson WR, et al. Ceftriaxone once daily for four weeks compared with ceftriaxone plus gentamicin once daily for two weeks for treatment of endocarditis due to penicillin-susceptible streptococci. *Clin Infect Dis.* 1998;27:1470–1474.

6. Tice AD. Outpatient parenteral antimicrobial therapy for osteomyelitis. *Infect Dis Clin North Am.* 1998;12:903–919.

7. Tice AD, Hoaglund PA, Shoultz DA. Risk factors and treatment outcomes in osteomyelitis. *J Antimicrob Chemother*. 2003;51:1261–1268.

8. Tice AD, Hoaglund PA, Shoultz DA. Outcomes of osteomyelitis among patients treated with outpatient parenteral antimicrobial therapy. *Am J Med*. 2003;114:723–728.

9. Nelson JD. Acute osteomyelitis in children. *Infect Dis Clin North Am*. 1990;4:513–522.

10. Gentry LO, Rodriguez GG. Oral ciprofloxacin compared with parenteral antibiotics in the treatment of osteomyelitis. *Antimicrob Agents Chemother*. 1990;34:40–43.

11. Tice AD. Ertapenem: a new opportunity for outpatient parenteral antimicrobial therapy. *J Antimicrob Chemother*. 2004;53(suppl 2):ii83–ii86.

12. Eron LJ, Marineau M, Baclig E, et al. The virtual hospital: treating acute infections in the home by telemedicine. *Hawaii Med J*. 2004;63:291–293.

13. Eron LJ, Passos S. Early discharge of infected patients through appropriate antibiotic use. *Arch Intern Med*. 2001;161:61–65.

14. Eron LJ, Lipsky BA, Low DE, et al. Managing skin and soft tissue infections: expert panel recommendations on key decision points. *J Antimicrob Chemother*. 2003;52(suppl 1):i3–i17.

15. Lindbeck G. Outpatient parenteral antibiotic therapy. Management of serious infections. Part II Amenable infections and models for delivery. Emergency department and urgent care center. *Hosp Pract*. 1993;28(suppl 2):44-47.

16. Arbeit RD, Maki D, Tally FP, et al. The safety and efficacy of daptomycin for the treatment of complicated skin and skin-structure infections. *Clin Infect Dis*. 2004;38:1673–1681.

17. Hardy WD. Home health care—an important component of the HIV patient care continuum. *Syntex*. 1991;1:1-5.

18. Wolf DL, Rodriguez CA, Mucci M, et al. Pharmacokinetics and renal effects of cidofovir with a reduced dose of probenecid in HIV-infected patients with cytomegalovirus retinitis. *J Clin Pharmacol*. 2003;43:43–51.

19. Saint-Leger E, Fillet AM, Malvy D, et al. [Efficacy of cidofovir in an HIV infected patient with an acyclovir and foscarnet resistant herpes simplex virus infection]. [Article in French]. *Ann Dermatol Venereol*. 2001;128:747–749.

20. Lazzarin A. Enfuvirtide: the first HIV fusion inhibitor. *Expert Opin Pharmacother*. 2005;6:453–464.

21. Freeman RB. Valganciclovir: oral prevention and treatment of cytomegalovirus in the immunocompromised host. *Expert Opin Pharmacother*. 2004;5:2007–2016.

22. Tice AD, Bonstell RP, Marsh PK, et al. Peripherally inserted central venous catheters for outpatient intravenous antibiotic therapy. *Infect Dis Clin Pract*. 1993;2:186–190.

23. Rucker RW, Harrison GM. Outpatient intravenous medications in the management of cystic fibrosis. *Pediatrics*. 1974;54:358–360.

24. Mandell LA, Bartlett JG, Dowell SF, et al. Update of practice guidelines for the management of community-acquired pneumonia in immunocompetent adults. *Clin Infect Dis*. 2003;37:1405–1433. Available at: www.journals.uchicago.edu/CID/journal/issues/v37n11/32441/32441.html. Accessed May 31, 2005.

25. American Thoracic Society. Guidelines for the management of adults with community-acquired pneumonia. *Am J Respir Crit Care Med*. 2001;163:1730–1754.

26. Ziss DR, Stowers A, Feild C. Community-acquired pneumonia: compliance with centers for Medicare and Medicaid services, national guidelines, and factors associated with outcome. *South Med J*. 2003;96:949–959.

27. Houck PM, Bratzler DW, Nsa W, et al. Timing of antibiotic administration and outcomes for Medicare patients hospitalized with community-acquired pneumonia. *Arch Intern Med*. 2004;164:637–644.

28. Fine MJ, Auble TE, Yealy DM, et al. A prediction rule to identify low-risk patients with community–acquired pneumonia. *N Engl J Med*. 1997;336:243–250.

29. Halm EA, Teirstein AS. Management of community-acquired pneumonia. *N Engl J Med.* 2002;347:2039–2045.

30. Metlay JP, Fine MJ. Testing strategies in the initial management of patients with community-acquired pneumonia. *Ann Intern Med.* 2003;138:109–118.

31. Tice AD. Community acquired pneumonia: recent insights into an old disease. *Infect Med.* 2003;20:352–356.

32. Fine MJ, Hough LJ, Medsger AR, et al. The hospital admission decision for patients with community-acquired pneumonia. *Arch Intern Med.* 1997;157:36–44.

33. Fine MJ, Medsger AR, Stone RA, et al. The hospital discharge decision for patients with community-acquired pneumonia. *Arch Intern Med.* 1997;157:47–56.

34. Ramirez JA. Processes of care for community-acquired pneumonia. *Infect Dis Clin North Am.* 2004;18:843–859.

35. Corwin P, Toop L, McGeoch G, et al. Randomised controlled trial of intravenous antibiotic treatment for cellulitis at home compared with hospital. *BMJ.* 2005;330:129.

36. Upton A, Ellis-Pegler RB, Woodhouse A. Outpatient parenteral antimicrobial therapy (OPAT): a review of experience at Auckland Hospital. *N Z Med J.* 2004;117:U1020.

37. Millar LK. Pyelonephritis. *Hosp Pract.* 1993;28(suppl 2):31–35.

38. McNeeley SG Jr. Pelvic inflammatory disease. *Curr Opin Obstet Gynecol.* 1992;4:682–686.

CHAPTER 4

Antimicrobial Selection for Outpatient Parenteral Antimicrobial Therapy

In selecting antimicrobials for outpatient parenteral antimicrobial therapy (OPAT), prescribing physicians must consider a number of factors in addition to those addressed in the hospital setting, including dosage schedule, long-term toxicity, and stability.[1]

Such considerations often may lead to the selection of different antimicrobials, different forms of traditional agents, different treatment schedules, and different modes of delivery than would be prescribed in the hospital for the same infection. Both the challenge of and the answers to antimicrobial selection for OPAT lie in the pharmacokinetics and pharmacodynamics of the common antimicrobial agents. The antimicrobials used by a variety of OPAT programs, as well as the most common infections treated, are listed in Table 4.1.[1]

Evidence of patient tolerance and a low incidence of toxic reactions are prerequisites for agents to be used outside the hospital, where patients cannot be as closely monitored. Finally, prescribing physicians and OPAT providers must be aware of the specific adverse effects associated with prolonged intravenous (IV) antimicrobial therapy. For example, the development of leukopenia or renal toxicity is not unusual after several weeks of apparently uneventful treatment in patients who gave no indication of a problem within the first week.

The less often a drug has to be administered, the more convenient therapy is for patients, thus facilitating compliance. Less frequent schedules also require less staff time in terms of training and troubleshooting. Many antimicrobial agents can be given once a day, and

Table 4.1. Infections Treated with Outpatient Parenteral Antimicrobial Therapy (OPAT) and the Antibiotics Used in 4 Studies or Sites

OPAT Network (1996–2002)[a]	Cleveland Clinic (1996–2000)[b]	Minneapolis Area (1978–1990)[c]	Children's Hospital San Diego (2000)[d]
Type of infection, ranked by frequency (% of OPAT courses)			
Skin and soft tissue (23)	Musculoskeletal	Cellulitis (15)	Bacteremia (16)
Osteomyelitis (15)	Infected devices	Osteomyelitis (13)	Pyelonephritis (13
Septic arthritis/bursitis (5)	Bacteremia	Late-stage Lyme disease (10)	Meningitis (13)
Bacteremia (5)	Intra-abdominal	Pyelonephritis and UTI (9)	Intra-abdominal (8)
Wound (4)	Skin and soft tissue	Septic arthritis (7)	Cellulitis (7)
Pneumonia (4)		Other (46)	Osteomyelitis (7)
Pyelonephritis (3)			Wound (7)
Antimicrobial, ranked by frequency of use (% of OPAT courses)			
Ceftriaxone (33)	Vancomycin (31)	—	Ceftriaxone (42)
Vancomycin (20)	Penicillins (20)	—	Meropenem (11)
Cefazolin (6)	Antivirals (12)	—	Cefazolin (11)
Oxacillin/nafcillin (5)	Cephalosporins (9)	—	Cefepime (6)
Aminoglycosides (5)	Aminoglycosides (5)	—	Ceftazidime (6)
Clincamycin (3)	Other β-lactams (4)	—	—

NOTE: UTI, urinary tract infaction.
[a] Data from OPAT Outcomes Registry (available at http://www.opat.com).
[b] Data from Susan Rahm, personal communication. Percentage of infections not recorded.
[c] Data from Williams, *Int J Antimicrob Agents*, 1995.
[d] Data from John Bradley, personal communication.
Adapted from Tice,[1] with permission.

some that require even less frequent administration are currently under development.[2] Antimicrobial stability is another consideration unique to home administration, which often requires storage of a drug for at least a few days after being mixed. Table 4.2 displays the parameters of the antimicrobials used for OPAT.[1]

■ *Pharmacokinetics*

Serum or plasma levels of drug are a result of the amount administered, volume of distribution, metabolism, and elimination from the body. The decline over time in blood levels, or the clearance rate of a drug, is measured by its half-life, defined as the time it takes for the amount of drug in the blood to fall by one half.[3,4] For most drugs, however, half-life remains constant regardless of how much drug is in the body.

The development of antimicrobials that can be administered infrequently has been a major factor contributing to the growth of OPAT.

Table 4.2.   Properties of Commonly Prescribed Antimicrobials at Various Temperatures

Drug	Half-life (h)	Phlebitis risk rating[b]	Optimal dilution (mg/mL[c])	Duration of stability, by storage temperature[a] −20°C	5°C	25°C
Acyclovir[d]	2–3.5	1	5	ND	37 d	>37 d
Amphotericin B	24–360	3	0.1	ND	35 d	5 d
Liposomal amphotericin B	24–360	2	4	ND	24 h	5 d
Amphotericin B lipid complex	24–360	2	1	ND	48 h	6 h
Ampicillin	1	2	30	ND	48 h	8 h
Ampicillin-sulbactam	1	2	20	ND	48 h	8 h
Caspofungin	>48	1	0.2–0.3	ND	24 h	1 d
Cefazolin	1–2	1	10–20	30 d	10 d	1 d
Cefoperazone	1.5–25	1	40	96 d	80 d	80 d
Ceftazidime	1.4–2	1	1–40	90 d	21 d	2 d
Ceftriaxone	5.4–10.9	1	10–40	180 d	10 d	3 d
Cefuroxime	1–2	1	5–10	30 d	180 d	1 d
Chloramphenicol	1.5–4	1	10–20	180 d	30 d	30 d
Clindamycin	2–3	1	6–12	56 d	32 d	16 d
Daptomycin	8.1	1	ND	ND	48 h	12 d
Doxycycline[e]	22–24	2	0.1–1	56 d	48 h	3 d
Erythromycin lactobionate	1.5–2	3	0.1–0.2	30 d	14 d	1 d
Ertapenem	4	2	20	ND	24 h	6 h
Ganciclovir	2.5–3.6	1	5	364 d	35 d	5 d
Gentamicin	2–3	1	0.6–1	30 d	30 d	30 d
Imipenem-cilastatin	0.8–1.3	2	2.5–5	ND	2 d	10 h
Linezolid	4.5	1	2	ND	ND	ND
Meropenem	1.5	1	5–20	ND	24 h	4 h
Nafcillin	0.5–1.5	3	2–40	90 d	3 d	1 d
Oxacillin	0.3–0.8	2	10–100	30 d	7 d	1 d
Penicillin G[f]	0.4–0.9	2	0.2	84 d	14 d	2 d
Quinupristin-dalfopristin	3/1	3	2	ND	54 h	5 h
TMP-SMZ[d]	8–11/10–13	2	8	ND	ND	6 h
Tobramycin	2–3	1	0.2–3.2	30 d	4 d	2 d
Vancomycin	4–6	2	5	63 d	63 d	7 d

NOTE: D, day(s); ND, no data; TMP-SMZ, trimethoprim-sulfamethoxazole.
[a] Data from Williams and Raymond, *Clin Pharmacokinet*, 1988.
[b] Degree of tendency to cause phlebitis: 1, mild; 2, moderate; 3, high.
[c] Optimal solutions may vary from saline to 5% dextrose, depending on the antibiotics.
[d] Should not be refrigerated.
[e] Protect from sunlight.
[f] Degradation products can form after a few hours.
Adapted from Tice et al.,[1] with permission.

If a medication must be given every 2, 4, or even 6 hours, OPAT is impractical without the use of a computerized ambulatory infusion pump (see Chapter 6). Pumps are expensive and may not be readily available; hence a patient may remain in the hospital. Drugs or delivery systems that require attention from a patient or caregiver every 8 hours or less often make OPAT more feasible. Twice-a-day dosage schedules can be handled easily by patient or caregiver, or, under some circumstances, by a visiting nurse. A once-daily or even less-frequent dosage schedule is very near the ideal for both home and infusion center administration.

Fortunately, there is now a multitude of antibiotics with long enough half-lives to permit treatment of most bacterial pathogens once daily. These include daptomycin, ceftriaxone, ertapenem, and metronidazole.

With continuous infusion, it takes about four half-lives before a drug reaches 90% of steady state; at which point, rate of elimination equals rate of infusion.[5] With intermittent dosing, drug concentration rises to a peak level and falls to a trough before the next dose is given. Thus, the β-lactam antimicrobials, because of their short half-lives and time-dependent killing, might best be given by continuous infusion.[5,6] Moreover, the β-lactams have only a brief postantibiotic effect (PAE), the time it takes bacteria to recover after antibiotic levels fall below the minimum inhibitory concentration (MIC).

The pharmaceutical industry is now investigating antimicrobials with particularly long half-lives, including teicoplanin, which may be used to treat diseases such as osteomyelitis with dosing only 3 times a week.[7] Dalbavancin is a lipoglycopeptide that may need to be dosed only once a week.[2] Cidofovir can be dosed every other week to treat cytomegalovirus.[8]

Because clearance is often slowed in patients with renal failure, some drugs, such as vancomycin and the aminoglycosides, need to be given only every few days. Given the deterioration of renal function with age, once-daily vancomycin may be an appropriate choice for elderly patients.

Some drugs may affect clearance as well. For example, probenecid has been used to delay renal elimination of β-lactam antibiotics such as penicillin, ampicillin, oxacillin, and the cephalosporins.

■ *Pharmacodynamics*

The advantages of once-a-day dosing have led to a review of the mechanisms of action (MOAs), or pharmacodynamics, of the aminoglycoside drugs, such as gentamicin, tobramycin, and amikacin. These agents, along with the quinolones and metronidazole, show marked concentration-dependent bactericidal activity (the higher the drug level, the faster and more extensive its killing effect) as well as a prolonged PAE.[6,9] Despite the aminoglycosides' relatively short 2- to 3-hour half-lives, both these characteristics suggested the possibility of optimal activity with longer intervals between doses.

Convenience and compliance aside, less-frequent dosing of aminoglycosides also appears to reduce the nephrotoxicity and possibly, the ototoxicity of the drugs.[9] In patients with normal renal function, a dose of gentamicin of 5 to 7 mg/kg every 24 hours should provide the desired trough level of less than 1.[10] Regular monitoring for renal and vestibular toxicity remains necessary.

However, the use of once-daily aminoglycoside therapy by pregnant women, children, elderly persons, and critically ill patients has not been fully evaluated. Once-daily dosing recommendations for patients with renal dysfunction, neutropenia, burns, liver disease, or endocarditis should be used with caution.[9]

Different MOAs

The antimicrobial agents can be divided into three categories based on their MOAs (Table 4.3).[10] The β-lactam antibiotics kill bacteria by interfering with the synthesis of microbial cell walls. Thus, once plasma concentration of a penicillin or cephalosporin falls below MIC, susceptible organisms begin to reproduce within a matter of a few hours.

Table 4.3.   Antimicrobial Pharmacodynamics and Dosing Regimens

Antibiotic	Pharmacodynamics	Regimen's Goal
Penicillins Cephalosporins Aztreonam	Bactericidal at minimal concentration; brief or no PAE	Maximize exposure time; keep serum levels >MIC
Daptomycin	Bactericidal against drug-resistant gram+ pathogens; significant PAE	Maximize exposure time; serum levels can fall below MIC
Carbapenems Vancomycin Macrolides	Bactericidal at minimal concentration; prolonged PAE	Maximize exposure time; serum levels can fall below MIC
Aminoglycosides Quinolones Metronidazole	Bactericidal at high concentration; prolonged PAE	Maximize concentration; attain peak serum level

NOTE: PAE = postantibiotic effect; MIC = minimum inhibitory concentration.
Adapted from Andes and Craig,[10] with permission.

Therefore, these agents are more appropriately given by continuous infusion than in intermittent doses. In fact, when penicillin was introduced in the 1940s, it was administered by continuous infusion; only later was it given intermittently, largely for the sake of convenience. Although intermittent infusion has been successful, we now have the technology to make continuous infusion much more convenient and, with the help of a pump, less expensive than intermittent infusion in terms of mixing and administration time for medical staff. Continuous infusion also may require less drug because there is no advantage to maintenance of levels greater than four times the MIC of susceptible organisms.[10] If an antimicrobial is to be administered by continuous infusion, an initial loading dose should be given.

A second category of antibacterial agents that are also effective at MIC includes the carbapenems, vancomycin, clindamycin, and the macrolides, as well as daptomycin, the first available agent from a new class of antibiotics, the cyclic lipopeptides.[11] These drugs have a more persistent PAE, however, so serum levels may be allowed to drop below MIC.

The third group of agents, which includes the aminoglycosides, is concentration-dependent. Because they inhibit protein and nucleic acid synthesis, they have long PAEs. The aim of the dosing regimen with these drugs is to attain high peak plasma levels to penetrate the bacterial cells. Once there is a high concentration within the bacteria, the extended PAE will prevent bacterial regrowth when tissue levels fall below MIC, thus making long dosing intervals possible.

■ Spectrum of Antimicrobial Activity

For a known infecting organism, a narrow-spectrum agent offers the advantage of specific activity plus the least disruption of the host's normal protective microbial flora. Moreover, the tendency of broad-spectrum antimicrobials to encourage multidrug-resistant bacteria is causing increasing concern worldwide.

Organism-specific agents are not always practical, however. When the microbiologic cause of an infection is not known in a febrile neutropenic patient, broad-spectrum therapy with one, two, and occasionally three antimicrobials may be necessary.[12] An abdominal abscess may present the need to cover a mixture of aerobic and anaerobic bacteria, as well as possible fungi.

Even after a specific pathogen has been identified, a broad-spectrum agent may be the appropriate choice. For example, both cefazolin and ceftriaxone may be active against an infecting organism, but only ceftriaxone offers central nervous system penetration and activity. A history of allergic reactions to antimicrobials may preclude use of a narrow-spectrum drug, such as penicillin or ampicillin.

Outpatient use of broad-spectrum antimicrobials may be appropriate if they are safer, better-tolerated, and more convenient to administer than narrow-spectrum agents. The risk of developing resistant organisms through the use of broad-spectrum agents is probably less in the community than in the hospital, where multidrug-resistant organisms are commonplace. If treatment courses are short-term and low-dose, selective pressures for resistance are limited in the outpatient setting.

■ *Stability*

In the hospital, IV medications are mixed on an as-needed basis with only a few hours between preparation and infusion. Therefore, the stability of an antimicrobial in solution is of no great concern. In the home, however, where patients may use premixed medication over intervals of 3 to 7 days, the stability factor is a primary consideration in choice of antimicrobial, method of delivery, or both. Stability information for many of the most commonly used antimicrobials is listed in Table 4.2.

The less often a medication has to be mixed and dispensed, the lower the cost in terms of staff time and use of a facility. Many home care companies try to dispense medications for a week at a time, a reasonable option for long-term OPAT if close clinical follow-up is available. Oxacillin, clindamycin, and vancomycin will remain stable after reconstitution for that long if stored in a refrigerator. An hour before infusion, they can be taken out and warmed to room temperature. Many agents listed will remain stable for 2 weeks or longer if frozen after mixing and allowed to rewarm before use, but the solution may take 8 hours to reach room temperature.

Antimicrobials with short half-lives (e.g., clindamycin, oxacillin, and vancomycin) can be used for intermittent infusion if the patient or caregiver is willing and able to learn how to reconstitute them just before use, usually through a simplified system, such as the ADD-Vantage® (Abbott Laboratories) or the Mini-Bag Plus® (Baxter Healthcare Corporation). These do-it-yourself options avoid the need for rewarming and save the cost of pharmacy mixing fees but do carry an added purchase cost.

Drugs that are stable at room or body temperature have advantages. They can be used in pumps that are set to run for several days without a change in medication reservoir. They are ideal for continuous infusion. Guidelines for sterility of infusion solutions may be found in the *United States Pharmacopeia*.

■ Safety

Antimicrobials proven to be safe and effective are preferred for OPAT. Those of questionable efficacy or toxicity should be administered only to carefully monitored inpatients. Because of the risk of anaphylaxis, it is standard practice to have personnel and equipment available to treat any adverse reaction when infusing or injecting the first dose of any antimicrobial in a medical facility. Although such reactions are unusual, the risk of fatality remains a major concern.

According to a study conducted by the OPIVITA Study Group of serious adverse events associated with OPAT, the incidence of delayed anaphylactoid reactions was approximately 0.5% and could occur up to 2 weeks after the initiation of therapy.[13] All such reactions were easily controlled with discontinuation of the medication and treatment with antihistamines. Approximately 5% of study patients had a drug reaction severe enough to warrant a change in antimicrobial agent.

Medical supervision of patients during administration of drugs associated with infusion-related anaphylactoid reactions, such as vancomycin, is also prudent. If the first dose is tolerated and rate of administration can be controlled with an infusion device, the medication can usually be given at home. The "red man" reaction to vancomycin, which occurs routinely with rapid administration, may vary from one patient to another but usually responds to antihistamine and a reduced infusion rate. The reaction also seems to lessen with time.

Antimicrobials with known toxicity also may not be suitable for home administration. For example, patients who need amphotericin B should be hospitalized for the first doses because of the potential for multiple and severe side effects.[13,14] Most patients then can be treated at an outpatient infusion center. (In some cities with large AIDS populations, even amphotericin B is routinely administered in the patient's home by a visiting nurse.[15]) Pentamidine, with its potential for leukopenia, hypoglycemia, and adverse reactions, also is not generally suitable for administration at home, where there is less margin for error and fewer resources for handling emergency situations. Table 4.4 displays the frequency of adverse effects serious enough to stop antimicrobial therapy, which differ according to the drug being administered.[1,16]

Table 4.4. Frequency of Adverse Effects Due to Intravenously Administered Antimicrobials Used for Outpatient Parenteral Antimicrobial Therapy (OPAT)

Variable	*Cfz*	*Ctz*	*Ctrx*	*Cm*	*Gm*	*Oxa*	*Naf*	*Van*	*Total*
				Antimicrobial					
Courses administered	781	456	4670	442	327	479	266	2881	10,302
Courses stopped early[a]									
n	32	16	136	34	26	40	26	144	454
%	4.1	3.6	2.9	7.7	8.0	8.4	9.8	5.0	4.4
Adverse effect, % of courses									
Rash	1.92	2.19	1.39	5.43	0.61	3.55	4.51	2.29	2.05
Diarrhea	0.38	0.00	0.45	0.90	0.00	0.63	0.38	0.07	0.33
Nausea	0.77	0.22	0.36	0.90	0.92	1.88	1.50	0.24	0.50
Renal	0.13	0.22	0.00	0.00	2.75	0.21	0.75	0.42	0.25
Leukopenia	0.26	0.22	0.09	0.23	0.00	0.42	2.26	0.21	0.21
Urticaria	0.51	0.00	0.19	0.45	0.00	0.21	0.00	0.49	0.29
Fever	0.00	0.44	0.41	0.45	0.00	0.42	0.75	1.18	0.59
Vestibular	0.00	0.00	0.00	0.00	3.06	0.00	0.00	0.10	0.13
Hepatic	0.13	0.00	0.04	0.00	0.00	1.04	0.38	0.00	0.09
Anaphylaxis	0.26	0.00	0.04	0.00	0.31	0.21	0.00	0.14	0.10
Anaphylactoid	0.26	0.00	0.02	0.00	0.00	0.00	0.00	0.07	0.05
Anemia	0.00	0.22	0.00	0.00	0.00	0.21	0.75	0.00	0.04

NOTE: Information gathered from the OPAT Outcomes Registry as of October 2002 (16). Cm. clindamycin; Ctrx, ceftriaxone; Ctz, ceftazidime; Cfz, cefazolin; Gm, gentamicin; Naf, nafcillin; Oxa, oxacillin; Van, vancomycin.
[a] Reactions recorded were only those serious enough to stop therapy with that antimicrobial. More than one reason for stopping therapy was rated in 20.1% of cases.
Adapted from Tice, et al.,[1] with permission.

■ *Laboratory Monitoring*

The guidelines displayed in Table 4.5 address the minimum frequency of monitoring for adverse reactions and toxicity. Additional studies may be needed for the determination of response to therapy. The table includes information from the OPAT Outcomes Registry, which indicates that 3% to 10% of antimicrobial courses are stopped prematurely because of adverse reactions.[1]

Renal function must be closely monitored with periodic tests in patients being treated with an aminoglycoside, ganciclovir, vancomycin, amphotericin B, or a β-lactam. More frequent tests should be made when two or more of these nephrotoxic agents are administered simultaneously.

Hepatitis is associated with nafcillin and fluconazole. Antimicrobials deplete the common bowel organisms and, in turn, vitamin K

Table 4.5.   Suggestions for Laboratory Parameters that Should be Monitored Weekly During Outpatient Parenteral Antimicrobial Therapy

Antimicrobial agent(s) by class	Frequency of testing, no. of times per week				Other
	Complete blood count[a]	Renal function tests[b]	Potassium levels	Liver enzyme levels	
Aminoglycosides (gentamicin, carbamycin, amikacin)	Once	Twice	—	—	Clinical monitoring (carbamycin amikacin) for vestibular and hearing dysfunction at each visit; serum concentrations as clinically indicated (see text)
β-Lactams (penicillins, cephalosporins, aztreonam, carbapenems)	Once	Once	—	—[c]	
Antipseudomonal penicillins	Once	Once	Once	—	
Fluoroquinolones	—	—	—	Once	
Miscellaneous					
Clindamycin	Once	Once	—	Once	
Daptomycin	Once	Once	—	Once	CPK at least weekly
Linezolid	Once	—	—	—	
Pentamidine	Twice	Twice	Twice	—	Blood glucose level daily; chemistry profile twice per week[d]
Quinupristin–dalfopristin	—	—	—	Once	Monitor for arthralgias
Trimethoprim-sulfamethoxazole	Once	Once	Once	—	
Vancomycin	Once	Once	—	—	Serum levels as clinically indicated
Antifungals					
Amphotericin B, including lipid formulations	Once	Twice	Twice	Once	Magnesium level once per week
Azole antifungal agents	Once	Once	—	Once	
Caspofungin	—	—	—	Once	
Antivirals					
Ganciclovir	Twice	Once	—	—	Magnesium level once per week
Acyclovir	Once	Once	—	—	Chemistry profile[d] with calcium and magnesium level once per week
Foscarnet	Once	Twice	Twice	Once	Urinalysis and chemistry profile[d] once per week
Cidofovir	Once	Once	Once	—	

NOTE: Frequencies are minimal criteria for patients with normal or stable renal function. Different criteria may apply for children.

[a] Should include a differential count of leukocytes and patient count.

[b] Renal function tests may include serum creatine and blood urea nitrogen levels and urinalysis. Trough levels appear to be the earliest indication of renal toxicity.

[c] Weekly liver enzyme tests with oxacillin, nafcillin, and carbapenems.

[d] A chemistry profile should include liver enzyme levels as well as electrolyte levels.

Adapted from Tice et al.,[1] with permission.

stores. Thus, prothrombin measurements should be considered, particularly if the patient is on anticoagulation therapy.

Leukopenia is an adverse effect commonly associated with the β-lactam antimicrobials and vancomycin,[17] but it does not occur within the first few days of therapy. Rather, the white cell count drops over a few weeks, during which patients seem otherwise stable and responsive to therapy. This phenomenon underscores the need for continued periodic laboratory testing during OPAT.

As new drugs become available, additional monitoring may be necessary, given the potential for adverse effects different from those of traditional antibiotics.

Patients vary in their ability to tolerate medication. Some may have a refractory "red man" syndrome despite all attempts to prevent its occurrence. Others may complain of bad taste, anorexia, lethargy, or other symptoms. Although not described in an antimicrobial's labeling, such subjective reactions do occur frequently enough to be addressed, even at times, to require a change of medication.

■ *Basic Criteria for OPAT Pharmaceuticals*

In the hospital, acquisition, storage, handling, preparation, and dispensing of all medications are carefully controlled and well documented. Well-established standards have evolved that guarantee the quality of drugs and the safety of patients receiving them. Safety and quality assurance standards are still being developed for the outpatient setting, however (see Chapter 7). It is critical, therefore, that minimal criteria be observed in acquiring, storing, preparing, and delivering the antimicrobial agents for OPAT.

The first basic principle is to purchase antimicrobials from suppliers who can guarantee their quality as well as ready access to additional supplies, whether from the manufacturer, a pharmaceutical wholesaler, or a mail-order company. After a drug's expiration date is checked, it should be stored under conditions recommended by the manufacturer; high temperatures and/or exposure to ultraviolet light can cause rapid deterioration of many pharmaceuticals.

Because an antimicrobial's cost may vary widely among suppliers, comparison shopping may result in significant savings. Group purchasing organizations may provide competitive pricing usually unavailable to smaller, independent programs.

Although it is possible to mix parenteral solutions in the absence of laminar air flow units, in most areas of the United States, pharmaceutical standards call for them. Specific vertical flow laminar hoods should be used for the preparation of chemotherapy solutions. Preferably, these hoods should be vented to the outside to prevent accidental exposure of the staff.

Once an antimicrobial solution has been prepared by a knowledgeable professional, it must be clearly labeled with drug name, patient name, date of mixing, expiration date, and storage requirements. Date and time of anticipated administration are also helpful and, in some cases, are required. The label should also contain information regarding type of infusion device and rate of administration. The initials of the pharmacist preparing the mixture and the pharmacy's name, address, and telephone number, as well as the prescription number and the prescribing physician's name, are required by State Boards of Pharmacy.

References

1. Tice AD, Rehm SJ, Dalovisio JR, et al. Practice guidelines for outpatient parenteral antimicrobial therapy. IDSA guidlines. *Clin Infect Dis.* 2004;38:1651–1672.

2. Dorr MB, Jabes D, Caveleri M, et al. Human pharmacokinetics and rationale for once-weekly dosing of dalbavancin, a semi-synthetic glycopeptide. *J Antimicrob Chemother.* 2005;55(suppl 2):ii25–ii30.

3. Holford NHG. Pharmacokinetics & pharmacodynamics: rational dosing & the time course of drug action. In: Katzung BG, ed. *Basic & Clinical Pharmacology.* 7th ed. Norwalk, CT: Appleton & Lange; 2003:35.

4. Wilkinson GR. Pharmacokinetics: the dynamics of drug absorption, distribution, and elimination. In: Hardman JG, Limbird LE, Gilman AG, eds. *Goodman and Gilman's The Pharmacological Basis of Therapeutics.* 10th ed. New York, NY: Pergamon Press; 2001:3–43.

5. Beam TR Jr, Brook I, Craig WA et al. Continuous vs. intermittent infusion of beta-lactam antibiotics: a potential advance. *Infect Med.* 1992;9(suppl B):1.

6. Craig WA. Basic pharmacodynamics of antibacterials with clinical applications to the use of β-lactams, glycopeptides, and linezolid. *Infect Dis Clin North Am.* 2003;17:479–501.

7. Graninger W, Wenisch C, Wiesenger E, et al. Experience with outpatient intravenous teicoplanin therapy for chronic osteomyelitis. *Eur J Clin Microbiol Infect Dis.* 1995;14:643–647.

8. Cundy KC, Petty BG, Flaherty J, et al. Clinical pharmacokinetics of cidofovir in human immunodeficiency virus-infected patients. *Antimicrob Agents Chemother.* 1995;39:1247–1252.

9. Dew RI, Sulsa G. Once-daily aminoglycoside treatment. *Infect Dis Clin Pract.* 1996;5:12–24.

10. Andes D, Craig WA. Pharmacokinetics and pharmacodynamics of outpatient intravenous antimicrobial therapy. *Infect Dis Clin North Am.* 1998;12:849–860.

11. Arbeit RD, Maki D, Tally FP, et al. The safety and efficacy of daptomycin for the treatment of complicated skin and skin-structure infections. *Clin Infect Dis.* 2004;38:1673–1681.

12. Talcott JA, Whalen A, Clark J, et al. Home antibiotic therapy for low-risk cancer patients with fever and neutropenia: a pilot study of 30 patients based on a validated prediction rule. *J Clin Oncol.* 1994;12:107–114.

13. Kunkel MJ, Tice AD, OPIVITA Study Group. Serious adverse events in outpatient parenteral antibiotic therapy: a prospective multicenter study [abstract]. *Proc Infect Dis Soc Am.* 1995:132.

14. Craven PC, Gremillion DH. Risk factors of ventricular fibrillation during rapid amphotericin B infusion. *Antimicrob Agents Chemother.* 1985;27:868–871.

15. Fernandez-Miera M, Farinas Alvarez MC, Hazas Feo MJ, et al. Intravenous amphotericin B at home, why not? [letter]. *Med Clin (Barc).* 1994;102:434–435.

16. Tice AD, Seibold G, Martinelli LP. Adverse effects with intravenous antibiotics with OPAT. Program and Abstracts of the 40th Annual meeting of the Infectious Diseases Society of America (IDSA); October 24–27, 2002; Chicago, IL. Abstract 59.

17. Tennican PO, Mortlock NJ, Tennican SP. Leukopenia and neutropenia: complications of outpatient IV antimicrobial therapy [abstract]. *Proc Infect Dis Soc Am.* 1992:17.

CHAPTER 5

Intravenous Access

The introduction and continuing improvement of safe, effective out-patient parenteral antimicrobial therapy (OPAT) parallel the rapid development of its key components, devices for intravenous (IV) access and delivery and the skilled specialists who place and control them in patient care (Table 5.1).[1]

Short peripheral IV catheters are flexible, more biocompatible, and less likely to perforate a vein or cause infiltration. They are appropriate for short-term OPAT, but not without limitations. Midline catheters last longer than short lines but are associated with late-onset phlebitis. Central venous tunneled catheters (CVTCs), such as the Hickman®, Broviac®, and Groshong®, allow provision of OPAT antimicrobials as well as parenteral nutrition, hemodialysis, and chemotherapy. Although most appropriate for weeks or months of therapy, these lines are more difficult and costly to insert. Peripherally inserted central venous catheters (PICCs) now provide convenient access to the superior vena cava with few complications and may be left in place for prolonged periods as access for both the delivery of medication and the drawing of blood. Finally, introduction of improved subcutaneous ports for venous access has solved a number of problems inherent in the use of CVTCs and PICCs for long-term OPAT.

■ *Peripheral Lines*

The original peripheral IV stainless steel needles have generally been replaced with biocompatible polyurethane and silicone, which

59

Table 5.1. Vascular Access Catheters

Type	Brand Name	Manufacturer
Peripheral	Protectiv* Plus™ Insyte™	Johnson & Johnson Medical Becton, Dickinson
Midline	First Midline V-Cath® L-Cath®	Becton, Dickinson HDC Corporation Luther Medical Products, Inc.
Central tunneled	Chemo-Cath® Groshong® Hickman® Broviac® C-TPN	HDC Corporation Bard Access Systems Bard Access Systems Bard Access Systems Cook Incorporated
Port	BardPort™ Life Port™ Port-A-Cath® Vital-Port® ChemoPort® CathLink 20™ Injection Port 3 PasPort® C-PICC® Groshong®	Bard Access Systems Strato/Infusaid SIMS Deltec, Inc. Cook Incorporated HDC Corporation Bard Access Systems EPS, Inc. Sims Deltec Incorporated Cook Incorporated Bard Access Systems
Peripherally inserted central	LifeVac® Per-Q-Cath® SoloPICC™ V-Cath®	Vygon Corporation GESCO SoloPak® Pharmaceuticals HDC Corporation

Adapted from Tice et al.,[1] with permission.

are flexible, easier to insert, and less likely to perforate a vein. These major improvements aside, however, peripheral lines are still associated with clotting, infiltration, and phlebitis within only a few days of insertion. Recommended standards, based on hospital rather than outpatient risks, are that lines be assessed daily and changed every 2 or 3 days.[2,3] Not all infusion programs comply with these standards, however. Many OPAT providers leave lines in for a week if patients are doing well.

These catheters should be irrigated or flushed regularly with saline solution and heparin to ensure maintenance of patency. A number of studies have supported the use of saline alone, and many OPAT providers are now doing so.[4,5] In the hospital, lines may be flushed every 8 hours, whereas home and outpatient protocols usually require the procedure only once a day after each dose—if there are few apparent patency problems. Nevertheless, short peripheral catheters are rarely used for more than 10 days. If a line becomes clotted or infiltration occurs between visits, the patient can simply pull it out and another can be inserted before the next dose. The catheters are also appropriate for outpatients who prefer to have a new IV line placed and removed after every infusion rather than have devices in their arms between visits. This approach may also be appropriate in situations of known or suspected drug abuse.

■ *Midline Catheters*

The midline catheter extends from the insertion site just distal to the antecubital fossa almost to the axillary vein. Designed for intermediate-duration therapy of 1 to 6 weeks, these 2- to 4-French catheters are introduced through an over–the-needle safety introducer or over a guidewire[1] (modified Seldinger technique) and may be advanced 7 to 10 inches.

The major advantages of the midline catheter over the conventional 1-inch peripheral catheter have been drug hemodilution and improved dwell time.[6] The vessel flow of the upper arm basilic and cephalic veins has been documented at 100 to 150 mL/min, as compared with 20 to 40 mL/min in those of the lower arm.[7] The increased flow dilutes a drug's pH and osmolarity, reducing the risk of phlebitis and infiltration. In addition, the midline catheter does not have to be removed as frequently as the conventional 1-inch peripheral catheter.[8,9]

Although the tip's placement just distal to the shoulder joint allows greater hemodilution of medications than short peripheral lines, this catheter is not suitable for total parenteral nutrition with glucose concentrations greater than 10%, with hyperosmolar solutions, or with chemotherapy, all of which require infusion into the vena cava for adequate dilution.

■ *Central Venous Catheters*

Long-term outpatient parenteral nutrition and renal dialysis require access to a large vein in order to provide adequate dilution and allow large volumes and high concentrations of infusate. Some antimicrobials, such as vancomycin, potassium penicillin, and amphotericin B should also be infused into a central vein to prevent peripheral phlebitis.

Central venous access is most commonly achieved via the subclavian vein, although the internal jugular and even the femoral veins offer good access to the vena cava. Most central lines are made of polyurethane, thus remain rigid during insertion and become more pliable when they reach body temperature. They are well tolerated and cause minimal inflammatory response. These catheters vary considerably in size and may contain two lumens for infusion of incompatible agents.

Hickman®, Broviac®, and Groshong® catheters are usually tunneled under the skin for 10 to 15 cm to create a barrier to infection and leave an exit site, usually on the anterior chest midway between nipple and sternum, that can be seen and accessed easily by patient or caregiver.[10] If cared for properly, the catheters carry a relatively small risk of infection. They can be left in place for years and can be used to draw blood as well as for infusion.

The major risks associated with subclavian lines are related to insertion. Even in experienced hands, pneumothorax, arterial bleeding or, occasionally, nerve injury may occur with a subclavian venipuncture and manipulation of the needle or catheter. Any of these could create a serious problem for patients with severe lung disease or coagulation disorders. Central line insertion is also costly, often more than several thousand dollars, including cost of the catheter and fees for the surgeon, anesthesiologist, and operating room (OR).

■ *Peripherally Inserted Central Catheters*

Improvements in plastic materials as well as catheter design have made possible the development of central lines that can be passed into the superior vena cava from a peripheral insertion site in the antecubital or basilic veins. The advantages of these PICCs include

- Insertion does not require a surgical procedure; an experienced nurse can insert a PICC in the infusion center (Figure 5.1)
- They provide access to a large vein
- They reduce risk of pneumothorax, hemothorax, or air embolism
- Insertion costs significantly less than surgical placement
- They are easily removed after completion of infusion therapy

In addition to their utility in long-term OPAT, PICCs are useful for patients who have had a chest wall injury, radical neck dissection,

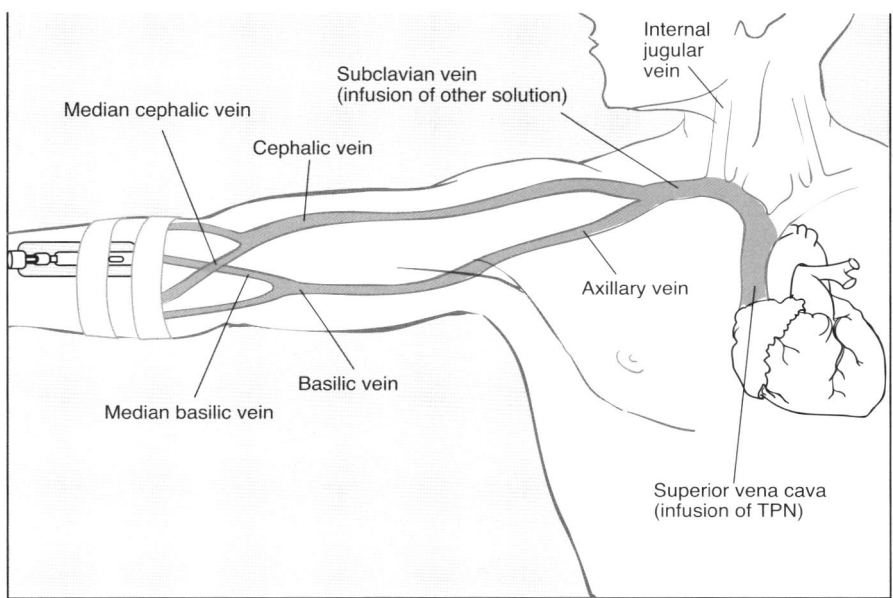

Figure 5.1. *Correct placement of a peripherally inserted central catheter (PICC). (Adapted from Phillips,[11] with permission.)*

bilateral mastectomy, postoperative radiation to the chest, or who are physically unable to undergo the surgical procedure required to place a subclavian line.

Made of polyurethane or silicone, PICCs are available in different sizes for insertion through 22- to 16-gauge needles (Table 5.2). Some lines come equipped with guidewires and some with breakaway needles, which can be removed easily to leave only a thin piece of flexible plastic in an antecubital vein. Several PICCs have double lumens. Some of the newer PICC lines have an antibacterial in the catheter sheath to prevent the lines from becoming infected.

The PICC is usually placed by a nurse specialist in the patient's hospital room or outpatient facility.[11,12] Interestingly, the success of PICCs in outpatient settings has resulted in their increased use in hospitals for patients with difficult vascular access or who are being given infusions of caustic medication. Because the catheters are not usually sutured in place and require sterile dressing changes, they should be managed by a nurse or physician.

Table 5.2. Peripherally Inserted Central Catheter (PICC) Lines

Company	Product Name	Materials	Lumens: Catheter Size	Introducer Type
Bard Access Systems	Per-Q-Cath®	Silicone	Single: 2 to 4 FR	Peel apart
Bard Access Systems	Groshong®	Silicone	Single: 3 to 4 FR	Peel apart
BD Medical Systems	First PICC™	Silicone	3 to 5 FR	Peel apart
BD Medical Systems	L-Cath™	Silicone or aliphatic polyurethane	Single: 2.6 to 5 FR Dual: 2.6 to 5 FR Pediatric/neonatal: 1.2 and 1.9 FR	Peel apart needle or peel apart sheath
BD Medical Systems	OneCath®	Aliphatic polyurethane	Single: 3.5 to 5.5 FR	Over-the-needle for needlestick prevention
Boston Scientific	Vaxcel® with PASV® Valve	Polyurethane	Single: 3 to 5 FR Dual: 4 to 6 FR	Peelable sheath
Boston Scientific	PASV®	Silicone	Single: 3 to 5 FR	Peelable sheath
Boston Scientific	Vaxcel®	Polyurethane	Single: 4 to 5 FR Dual: 5 to 6 FR	Peelable sheath
Cook, Inc.	C-PICCs	Silicone	Single: 3 to 5 FR	Peel-Away® sheath
Smiths Medical	CliniCath®	Polyurethane	Single: 2 to 5 FR Dual: 4 to 5 FR	Safety micro-introducer or sheath introducer
HDC Corporation	V-Cath® PICC	Silicone	Single: 2 to 4.5 FR Single: 2 to 4.5 FR	Break-away needle or Safe-T-Peel® sheath
Vygon Corporation	LifeVac® PICC	Silicone	3 to 5 FR	*SN 17G–PS 18G *SN 16G–PS 17G *SN 14G–PS 16G

Adapted from Tice et al.,[1] with permission.

Some PICC lines cause an initial sterile phlebitis, which progresses up the arm for 5 to 10 cm from the insertion site within a day or two after placement. This local reaction does not appear to be caused by infection and responds well, within a few days, to hot packs plus anti-inflammatory agents. Prophylactic ibuprofen or coumadin may be of some value in preventing this reaction.

Infection seems to be associated less often with peripherally inserted than with subclavian lines. According to one study, septic phlebitis occurred in only 0.7% of more than 600 patients with bacteremia,[13] which compared favorably with a bloodstream infection rate of 1% to 5% associated with other central lines.[14] Mechanical problems are more common with PICCS, however, with nearly 10% of lines removed early because of dislodgement, leakage, or occlusion.

A recent survey of infectious disease specialists documented the high frequency of line-related infectious as well as noninfectious complications with PICC lines during OPAT.[15] This information clearly demonstrates the need for ongoing medical expertise and follow-up. A recent article has also suggested a registry for PICC providers which would track their outcomes compared with other programs.[16]

When a PICC is placed, the catheter length should be recorded and checked again when it is removed.[1] A chest radiograph should be performed after placement to confirm the position of the catheter tip.[17-20] Instructions for PICC use and maintenance must be clear and detailed. The dressing over the exit site should be changed by a trained nurse at least weekly, more often if necessary, to prevent infection or dislodgement of the catheter, especially if the PICC is not sutured in place. Moreover, excessive pressure during infusions or flushing may rupture these catheters at the hub. A major disadvantage for patients is the fact that the PICC line should not get wet, so bathing, swimming, hot tubs, and hot weather pose a threat to the line's long-term viability.

Some PICCs have been left in place for more than a year. Their low reactivity with the intima is documented by the fact that after removal of one line, the same vein has been used repeatedly.[12]

Peripherally inserted central venous catheters are more expensive than peripheral catheters, but their use can result in considerable savings in terms of nursing time and material costs of peripheral line restarts. Thus, PICCs may compare quite favorably on a cost basis, particularly for self- and caregiver-administration of OPAT, which would require costly nurse-specialist home visits to address peripheral line problems. After initial placement of a PICC, a patient with osteomyelitis, for example, can be treated for 6 weeks without undergoing another venipuncture.

Although PICCs are often used for blood sampling as an alternative to venipuncture, the procedure carries a hypothetical risk of catheter occlusion caused by blood remaining in the catheter, and the practice is not supported by PICC manufacturers. However, a recent study of children with 3-French PICC catheters in place compared the catheter occlusion rate in patients whose catheters were used for blood sampling and those whose were not.[21] A higher occlusion rate in the blood sampling group did not reach statistical significance, and the investigators concluded that blood sampling is feasible and effective through these PICCs. Moreover, the practice was not associated with a significant increase in infection or mechanical complication rates.

■ Ports

The implanted port solves some of the problems associated with long-term or intermittent OPAT using tunneled central venous catheters (CVCs) and PICCs. It requires little maintenance between infusions, is safely concealed beneath the patient's skin, is impervious to water, and provides an additional barrier to infection as well.

Although a variety of ports are available from several different manufacturers, all share three basic components.[1] The portal body is a solid-cast chamber implanted in a subcutaneous pocket. Constructed of surgical stainless steel, titanium, plastic polymers, or some combination of the three, it provides sites for both introduction of the infusion device and attachment of the venous catheter.

The portal septum, which is made of highly compressed silicone material, provides a seal between the vascular system and the outside environment. The septum will generally remain intact, without leaking, after being breached from 1000 to 2000 times with the Huber needle, which is angled and has a curved tip to prevent its removing a plug of plastic with each insertion.

The portal catheter, which is made of silicone or polymer, may be placed in the venous, arterial, intraspinal, or peritoneal areas. The catheter is attached to the portal body either permanently or by a locking mechanism. Either a cutdown or percutaneous vascular access technique is used for venous catheter placement, which requires the skill and expertise of a surgeon and is usually done in the OR under general anesthesia.

A more recently introduced peripheral venous port has simplified the insertion procedure.[22] The subcutaneous port can be placed in the forearm with the associated catheter positioned in the central circulation via the basilic, median, antecubital, or cephalic vein (Figure 5.2). The entire cost of placing a peripheral port may be less than that of a central line placed in the OR.

■ *Catheter Care*

Care of IV lines and catheters has been standardized for most hospital settings, with guidelines set forth by the Centers for Disease Control and Prevention as well as the Intravenous Nurses Society.[8,23] Care in the outpatient setting is not as well standardized, however. Patients, environment, and other practical issues are different and have led to a wide variety of procedures and protocols (Table 5.3). Protocols for exit site dressing changes remain unstandardized as well, even controversial. A number of cleansing agents are available. Alcohol removes skin oils and squamous skin cells but has no residual antimicrobial activity. Povidone-iodine provides sustained release of free iodine, which has an antibacterial and antifungal effect that decreases as it dries. Chlorhexidine has a residual antibacterial and antifungal effect that lasts up to several hours after application. Regardless of the agent used, the area should be cleaned thoroughly with friction, working outward from the exit site in a circular motion; the area should be completely dry before a new dressing is applied.

■ *Support Products*

A number of products have been developed to support safe, reliable venous access in the outpatient setting, including prefilled flush kits for both peripheral and CVCs. Although they are significantly more expensive than do-it-yourself vials and syringes, the kits afford a measure of convenience and safety through reduction in required manipulations and tasks for patient or caregiver. For home care patients with poor vision, limited manual dexterity, or compromised short-term memory, they may prove to be the only way to ensure compliance with flushing protocols.

Repair kits are available for many brands of CVC and PICC lines. With one of these kits, an experienced nurse or physician can seal a hole or tear in a catheter in the outpatient clinic or patient's home. A number of special attachment systems are available to prevent tubing and needles from becoming disconnected accidentally. Special

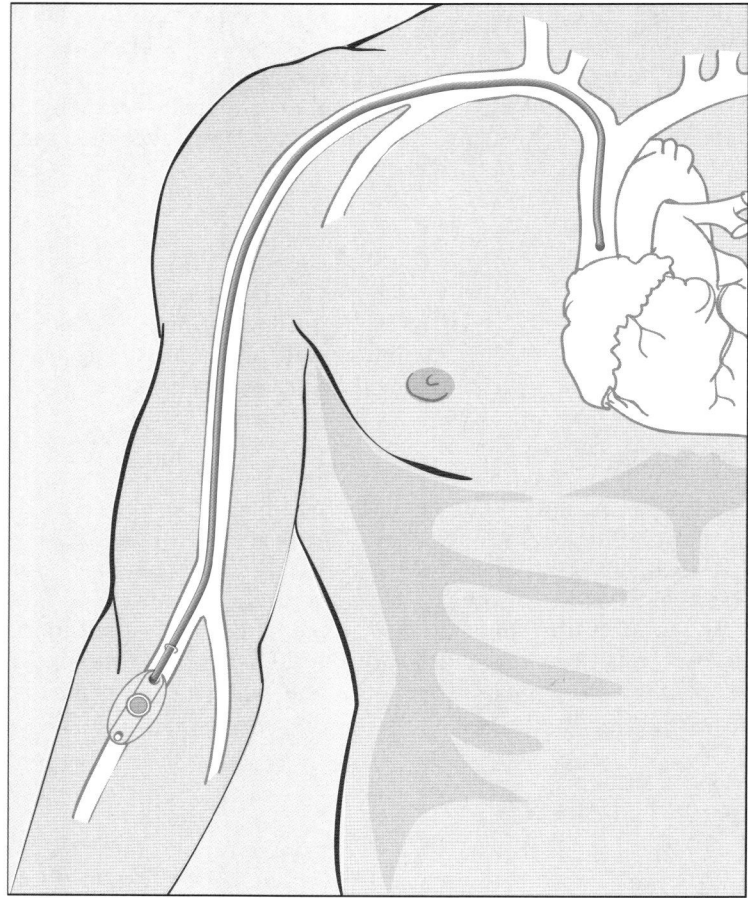

Figure 5.2. *Correct placement of a peripheral port and catheter. (Courtesy of Pharmacia Deltec, Inc., St. Paul, Minnesota.)*

clips are available to occlude catheters without damaging the tubing. Antibacterial cuffs placed at the insertion site discourage bacterial growth. Antibiotic- or silver-impregnated catheters that discourage bacterial growth are also available.

Regulations and guidelines regarding bloodborne pathogens promulgated by the U.S. Occupational Safety and Health Administration (OSHA)[24] have spurred the development of a number of so-called needleless or recessed needle systems to replace exposed hypodermic

Table 5.3. Central Venous Catheter Care: Irrigation and Dressings

Catheter Type	Flushing Frequency	Flushing Volumes Saline	Flushing Volumes Heparin	Dressing Changes and Frequency	When in Use
Peripheral	Q 8–24 hours and prn	1–10 ml	See #1 below	With restart and prn	SAS*
Midline	Q 8–24 hours and prn	5–10 ml	See #1 below	Weekly and prn	SAS
Non-tunneled	Q 8–24 hours and prn	5–10 ml	See #1 below	Weekly and prn Transparent	SAS
Tunneled and PICCs	Q 8–24 hours and prn	10 ml	See #1 below	Weekly and prn Transparent	SAS
Catheters with built in valves	Q week and prn	10 ml	See #1 below	Weekly and prn Transparent	SAS for all types
Implanted ports Accessed Deaccessed	Q 24 hours and prn Q month	10 ml 20 ml	100u/ml, 2.5–5.0ml with weekly reaccess and prn	With weekly reaccess and prn Use non-coring needles for accessing	SAS SAS

[1]A PRN heparin (10 u/ml, 5ml) order is helpful if the catheter becomes sluggish to irrigation.

*SAS, Saline–Administration–Saline

Adapted from Regional Infusion Leadership Council, Spokane, Washington, with permission.

needles in IV lines.[25,26] These may be particularly helpful in preventing the spread of bloodborne pathogens to health care workers.

In summary, OPAT has been made possible and continues to be improved and facilitated by the development of increasingly safe, reliable vascular access, through a variety of new catheters, ports, and innovative support products.

References

1. Tice AD. Outpatient Intravenous Therapy Source Book. Tacoma, WA: OPIT Source Book. 2004. Available at: www.opitsourcebook.com. Accessed June 28, 2005.

2. Tice AD, Rehm SJ, Dalovisio JR, et al. Practice guidelines for outpatient parenteral antimicrobial therapy. IDSA guidlines. *Clin Infect Dis.* 2004;38:1651–1672.

3. Infusion Nurses Society. Infusion nursing standards of practice. *J Intraven Nurs.* 2000;23(suppl 6):S1–S88.

4. ASHP therapeutic position statement on the institutional use of 0.9% sodium chloride injection to maintain patency of peripheral indwelling intermittent infusion devices. *Am J Hosp Pharm.* 1994;51:1572–1574.

5. Goode CJ, Titler M, Rakel B, et al. A meta-analysis of effects of heparin flush and saline flush: quality and cost implications. *Nurs Res.* 1991;40:324–330.

6. Anderson NR. Midline catheters: the middle ground of intravenous therapy administration. *J Infus Nurs.* 2004;27:313–321.

7. Peripherally inserted central venous and midline catheters defining a vascular access early assessment program for advanced practice. *Bard Access Systems.* 2002:44–82.

8. O'Grady NP, Alexander M, Dellinger EP, et al. Guidelines for the prevention of intravascular catheter-related infections. Centers for Disease Control and Prevention. *MMWR Recomm Rep.* 2002;51(RR–10):1–29.

9. Intravenous Nurses Society. Infusion nursing standards of practice. *J Intraven Nurs.* 2000;23(6S).

10. McCluskey MM. Antineoplastic therapy. In: Weinstein SM, ed. *Plumer's Principles and Practice of Intravenous Therapy.* 7th ed. Philadelphia, PA: JB Lippincott; 2001; 474–547.

11. Phillips LD. *Manual of I.V. Therapeutics.* 4th ed. Philadelphia, PA: FA Davis; 2005.

12. Mortlock N. Intravenous therapy in the acute care setting. In: Hankins J, Lonsway RA, Hendrick C, Perdue M, eds. *Infusion Therapy in Clinical Practice.* 2nd ed. Philadelphia, Pa: WB Saunders; 2001:469–500.

13. Kunkel MJ, Tice AD, OPIVITA Study Group. Serious adverse events in outpatient parenteral antibiotic therapy: a prospective multicenter study [abstract]. *Proc Infect Dis Soc Am.* 1995:132.

14. Maki DG. Infections caused by intravascular devices used for infusion therapy: pathogenesis, prevention, management. In: Bisno AL, Waldvogel FA, eds. *Infections Associated with Indwelling Medical Devices.* 2nd ed. Washington, DC: American Society for Microbiology; 1994:155–212.

15. Strausbaugh LJ, Tice AD, Martinelli OP, et al. Experience of infectious diseases consultants with outpatient parenteral antimicrobial therapy: results of an emerging infections network service. Poster presented at: 15th Annual Scientific Meeting of the Society for Healthcare Epidemiology of America (SHEA); April 9–12, 2005; Los Angeles, CA.

16. Costa N. You are only as good as your data: developing an electronic PICC database. *J Assoc Vasc Access.* 2005;10:34–42.

17. Racadio JM, Doellman DA, Johnson ND, et al. Pediatric peripherally inserted central catheters: complication rates related to catheter tip location. *Pediatrics*. 2001;107:E28.

18. Allen AW, Megargell JL, Brown DB, et al. Venous thrombosis associated with the placement of peripherally inserted central catheters. *J Vasc Interv Radiol*. 2000;11:1309–1314.

19. Harako ME, Nguyen TH, Cohen AJ. Optimizing the patient positioning for PICC line tip determination. *Emerg Radiol*. 2004;10:186–189.

20. James L, Bledsoe L , Hadaway LC. A retrospective look at tip location and complications of peripherally inserted central catheter lines. *J Intraven Nurs*. 1993;16:104–109.

21. Knue M, Doellman D, Rabin K, et al. The efficacy and safety of blood sampling through peripherally inserted central catheter devices in children. *J Infus Nurs*. 2005;28:30–35.

22. Finney R, Albrink MH, Hart MG, et al. A cost-effective peripheral venous port system placed at the bedside. *J Surg Res*. 1992;53:17–19.

23. Mermel LA, Farr BM, Sheretz RJ, et al. Guidelines for the management of intravascular catheter-related infections. *J Intraven Nurs*. 2001;24:180–205.

24. Occupational Safety and Health Administration. *Model Exposure Control Plan for Home Care: A Guide for Hospice-Home Agencies on the Bloodborne Pathogens Standards*. Washington, DC: U.S. Government Printing Office; 1994.

25. Mendelson MG, Short LJ, Schechter CB, et al. Study of a needleless intermittent intravenous-access system for peripheral infusions: analysis of staff, patient, and institutional outcomes. *Infect Control Hosp Epidemiol*. 1998;19:401–406.

26. Danzig LE, Short LJ. Collins K, et al. Bloodstream infections associated with a needleless intravenous infusion system in patients receiving home infusion therapy. *JAMA*. 1995;273:1862–1864.

CHAPTER 6

Infusion Devices

The classic gravity drip system can be used by a nurse to deliver outpatient parenteral antimicrobial therapy (OPAT) in an infusion center or at home. In fact, patients can self-administer medications with this system, although training is detailed and often lengthy. Patients must have fine motor coordination and strength as well as the mental and visual acuity to monitor infusion rate. However, this system requires tethering to a gravity bag and, for ambulatory patients, dragging around the whole cumbersome unit.

Although the gravity drip system is still used for intermittent infusion in patients' homes, syringe pumps can provide the same or better reliability at equal or lower cost and with less time required for patient training. Of additional interest are the computerized ambulatory infusion pumps that can extend the benefits of OPAT to patients otherwise ineligible for intravenous (IV) antimicrobial treatment outside the hospital.

Thanks to a variety of modern technological advances, such as microelectronics and precision plastic manufacturing, many parenteral fluids and medications can now be administered by ambulatory infusion pumps. Originally developed to control the administration of IV drugs highly sensitive to rate and dosage changes in hospital intensive care units, infusion devices or pumps are currently used throughout the hospital to administer medications safely without constant nursing supervision. Further adaptation to the demands of outpatient therapy has resulted in an increasing array of smaller, lighter, more precise, reliable devices, some with built-in alarms. The major pump manufacturers are listed in Appendix 6A.

There is also interest in the continuous infusion of antibiotics, particularly β-lactams. Their activity is not concentration-dependent, thus may pose a risk when levels fall below the minimum inhibitory concentration.[1] Infusion pumps offer the advantage of programming, which may be a clinical as well as a staff time benefit.

■ *Syringe Pumps*

With these devices, fluid from the drug reservoir—the syringe—is propelled by forcing the plunger, or piston, into the syringe barrel. Syringe pumps are usually battery driven, although other power sources include a spring-loaded system and even an elastic band.[2] The prefilled syringe is clipped into the pump, which can be adjusted for different infusion rates, ranging from approximately 0.10 to 300 mL/h (Figure 6.1). If a large number of doses is required, several syringes can be filled, capped, and stored for later use. Syringe volumes may vary from 1 to 100 mL.[2,3] The pump's accuracy is usually

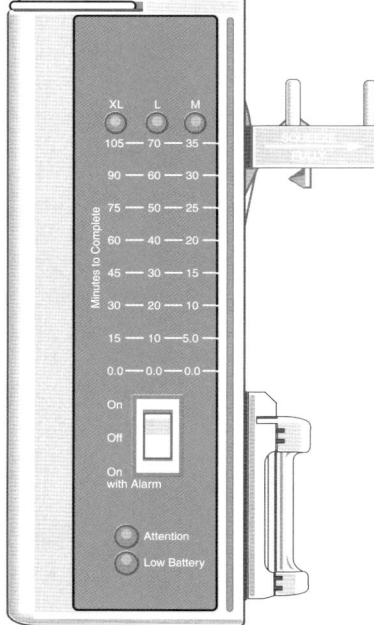

Figure 6.1. *Syringe pumps are useful for infusions of small doses of high-potency drugs. Prefilled syringes are clipped into the pump, which can be adjusted for different infusion rates.*

within 5%, which is acceptable for single-dose, short-term adminis-trations.[3-5] Syringe pumps can be portable and are connected to lines with microbore tubing.

Although training in the use of a syringe pump is simplified, patients still must learn to flush lines and correctly connect and disconnect tubing. Furthermore, dilution volume limitations may necessitate placement of a central venous catheter to prevent chemical phlebitis.

■ *Elastomeric Infusers*

Elastomeric infusion devices have a balloon reservoir that is pres-surized when filled with fluid.[2,6,7] Deflation and, in turn, infusion rates are controlled by specialized tubing. Pumps vary in size from 50 to 500 mL, with flow rates ranging from 0.5 to 200 mL/h. Delivery rate is not as precise as that of the syringe pump, with potential vari-ations as great as 15%. Pumps are disposable, with a new container used for each dose.

The pumps, commonly referred to as "home pumps," "baby bot-tles," "grenades," or "elastomerics," are lightweight and unobtrusive and can be stored in the refrigerator. They are ideal for children and helpful for patients who must work, go to school, or care for children while receiving an infusion. Elastomeric pumps are limited by low delivery pressure, which may result in inadequate flow through a crimped line or a partial occlusion. Flow rate may decrease or increase as a patient changes arm position, even if a peripherally inserted central venous catheter (PICC) line is in place. The system has no alarm mechanism. Some pumps have been known to rupture or leak if frozen. Most must be taken out of a refrigerator 4 to 8 hours before infusion to ensure accurate flow rate. Although special elas-tomeric pumps for administration of chemotherapy at home have been developed, because they are not electronic, they are not reim-bursable under current Medicare reimbursement guidelines.

■ *Computerized Infusion Devices*

The application of computer technology to infusion devices has led to remarkable advances. Pumps are now available that can administer up to four different solutions at different rates and inter-vals, from continuous infusion to circadian rhythm dosing (Figure 6.2).[3] They can provide reliability and a precision of administration seldom matched in the hospital, where nurses still administer and supervise parenteral therapy yet have many other patient care tasks to perform at the same time.

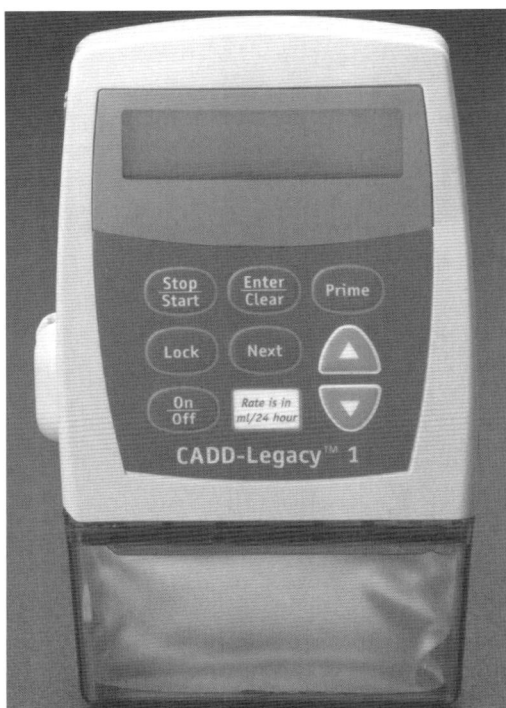

Figure 6.2.   *Programmable pumps can administer a number of different solutions at different rates and intervals.*

These pumps can be programmed for either intermittent or continuous infusion of antibiotics, and at least one delivers preflushing or postflushing of lines or both. Some can be adapted to volumes as large as 10 L and can be programmed to administer medications over a week's time. Rates of infusion can be adjusted from 0.10 to 500 mL/h.

Many patients previously considered ineligible for self-administration of antimicrobials in the home can be safely and effectively treated with these pumps. Among such patients are those who

- Require frequent (4- to 6-hour) dosing or even continuous infusion
- Have impaired manual dexterity or cognitive function
- Are unwilling or unable to learn the necessary techniques for self-administration
- Have an aversion to needles
- Lack a support person at home
- Are immunologically compromised (because the pump reduces the number of times the cannula has to be manipulated)

Although the pumps can be used to infuse medication through peripheral veins, they are more reliable and carry less risk of drug-related phlebitis when used with a centrally placed line or a PICC.

The power for the electronic pumps is provided by rechargeable battery packs or disposable alkaline batteries. Battery life varies with type of infusion but can last from 24 hours to several days. All pumps require their own brand of disposable IV tubing sets and special cartridges.

These devices allow patients receiving long-term OPAT to continue their daily activities with a portable, safe, effective, and discreet delivery system. The portable pumps weigh as little as 6 oz and as much as 37 oz. Like all sophisticated equipment, these devices have the potential to malfunction; errors may occur if a pump is programmed incorrectly, if the batteries run down, or if infusion cartridges are not placed properly. With multidose cassettes, a mistake in drug dose or concentration may be repeated many times before the error is detected.

There have been several recalls of pumps because of faulty performance.[4] Careful maintenance is a critical factor when pumps are to be reused.

Some pumps are equipped with alarms that signal an occlusion in the line, an up-line occlusion, a low reservoir, a weak battery, or a missed dose, as well as a lockout feature to prevent tampering.[7]

A major drawback to electronic pumps is their cost, which may be $2,000 to $6,000 per unit. Of course, the expense may be justified if the alternative is hospitalization or frequent visits of a nurse specialist to the patient's home. Another significant disadvantage of the pumps lies in the fact that some medications, such as ampicillin and imipenem, are not stable at room temperature long enough for administration via a 24-hour cassette.

■ *Selecting a Pump*

The two primary pump requirements for the four major home infusion therapies—antiinfective, analgesic, antineoplastic, and total parenteral nutrition/hydration—are flow range and reservoir capacity (Table 6.1).[1] Antimicrobial regimens usually consist of intermittent IV infusions of agents dissolved in 10 to 250 mL of solution. Doses generally are infused at rates of 50 to 100 mL/h over a period of 30 minutes to 3 hours, up to four times a day. Accuracy and continuity of flow usually are not very critical with antimicrobial therapy; infusion of the complete dose within a reasonable period is often adequate.

Table 6.1.   Primary Pump Requirements for Major Infusion Therapies

	Therapy				
	Antimicrobials	Analgesia—Continuous and Patient Controlled (PCA)	Chemotherapy	Total Parenteral Nutrition (TPN)	Hydration
Maximum reported range of flows, mL/hr[a]	5–250	0.4–10[b]	0.2–10	50–400	40–400
Maximum reported range of volumes delivered, mL[a]	10–250	10–250[b]	10–250	1000–3000	500–2000
Intermittent delivery	Essential[c]	Not necessary	Not necessary	See note d	See note d
Patient-controlled bolusing	Not necessary	Essential for PCA	May be useful for multidrug ancillary infusions (for example, antiemetics)	Not necessary	Not necessary
Ramping/circadian flow	Not necessary	Circadian rarely necessary	Circadian sometimes necessary	See note e	Not necessary
Other considerations	KVO and programmable loading dose may be useful	Tamper resistant/evident, programming in mass units and bolus history desirable	Accuracy		

[a]Many regimens may require less capability than the maximum reported ranges indicated.
[b]IV delivery only; subcutaneous flow range is 0.1–5.0 mL/hr with 10–25 mL reservoir capacity.
[c]Intermittent delivery can be accomplished with syringe drivers or elastomeric pumps that run out after delivering each dose or with programmable pumps that can deliver multiple doses from a single reservoir.
[d]TPN and hydration regimens generally are programmed by specifying volume to be infused and the time over which it is to be delivered. Restart of intermittent regimens generally is manual.
[e]Flow ramping is essential for intermittent TPN regimens but not necessary for continuous (24-hour) regimens.
Adapted from Ritter HTM III, Sacks ES. Home infusion devices. In: Conners RB, Winters RW, eds. Home Infusion: Current Status and Future Trends. Chicago: Health Forum. 1995, with permission.

Catheter patency between infusions, which may be required with intermittent delivery to a central venous line, is most conveniently accomplished by using a pump that reverts to a KVO (keep vein open) rate at the end of every infusion. Manual saline or heparin flush is necessary with most ambulatory infusion devices because few have automated catheter maintenance mechanisms.

With the increasing acceptance of outpatient care as a safe, cost-effective, even preferred alternative to hospitalization for many patients, new and improved infusion devices designed specifically for OPAT have been and will continue to be introduced. Moreover, as more patients are treated primarily in or discharged early to outpatient settings, it seems likely that the cost of these devices will gradually decrease.

References

1. Andes D, Craig WA. Pharmacokinetics and pharmacodynamics of outpatient intravenous antimicrobial therapy. *Infect Dis Clin North Am.* 1998;12:849–860.

2. Mortlock N. Intravenous therapy in the alternative care setting. In: Hankins J, Lonsway RA, Hendrick C, Perdue M, eds. *Infusion Therapy in Clinical Practice.* 2nd ed. Philadelphia, Pa: WB Saunders; 2001:535–560.

3. Mortlock NJ, Schleis TG. Outpatient parenteral antimicrobial therapy technology. *Infect Dis Clin North Am.* 1998;12:861–878.

4. Saladow J. Making sense of the options: infusion pumps for alternate site therapy. *Infusion.* 1995; 1(7, pt I):17–29;1(10, pt II):9–21.

5. Tice AD. *Outpatient Intravenous Therapy Source Book.* Tacoma, WA: OPIT Source Book, 2005. Available at: www.opitsourcebook.com. Accessed May 12, 2005.

6. Rich DS. Evaluation of a disposable, elastomeric infusion device in the home environment. *Am J Hosp Pharm.* 1992;49:1712–1716.

7. Rosenthal K. The new look of I.V. therapy. Improvements to existing products and technology enhance patient care, satisfaction, and outcomes. *Nurs Manage.* 2004;35:66–70.

Appendix 6A.   Infusion Device Manufacturers

3M Health Care	3M Center, Bldg. 275-4E-01 St. Paul, MN 55144 Phone: 800-228-3957 www.3M.com/healthcare
Alaris® Medical Systems	10221 Wateridge Circle San Diego, CA 92121-2772 Phone: 858-458-7524 www.alarismed.com/na
Bard Access Systems	5425 W. Amelia Earhart Drive Salt Lake City, UT 80116 Phone: 800-545-0890 www.bardaccess.com
Baxa Corporation	14445 Grasslands Drive Englewood, CO 80122-7062 Phone: 800-567-2292 www.baxa.com
Baxter Healthcare Corporation	Medication Delivery Division Rte 120 and Wilson Road Round Lake, IL 60073 Phone: 800-933-0303 www.baxter.com
B. Braun Medical Inc.	824 Twelfth Avenue Bethlehem, PA 18018-0027 Phone: 800-227-2862 www.bbraunusa.com
BD Medical Systems (Vascular Access Catheters)	9450 South State Street Sandy, UT 84070 Phone: 801-565-2300 www.bd.com/infusion
Boston Scientific	One Boston Scientific Place Natick, MA 01760 Phone: 800-225-3238 www.bostonscientific.com
Cook, Inc.	PO Box 489 Bloomington, IN 47402 Phone: 800-457-4500 www.cookgroup.com
Disetronic Medical Systems	5151 Program Avenue St. Paul, MN 55112 Phone: 763-795-5200 www.disetronic-usa.com
Excelsior Medical Corporation	1923 Heck Ave. Neptune, NJ 07753 Phone: 732-776-7525 www.excelsiormedical.com
HDC Corporation	628 Gibraltar Court Militas, CA 95035 Phone: 800-227-8162 www.hdccorp.com

Appendix 6A. *(Continued)*

Hospira World Wide Inc. (Formerly Abbott Laboratories Vascular Access)	275 North Field Drive BLDG HI,m Dept. PA 83 Lake Forest, IL 60045 www.hospira.com
ICU Medical	951 Calle Amanecer San Clemente, CA 92673 Phone: 800-824-7890 or 949-366-2183 www.icumed.com
I-Flow Corporation	20202 Windrow Drive Lake Forest, CA 92630 Phone: 800-448-3569 www.iflo.com
Medi-Dose, Inc./EPS, Inc.	Milton Building 70 Industrial Drive Ivyland, PA 18974 Phone: 800-523-8966 or 215-396-8600 www.medidose.com
Repro-Med Systems, Inc.	24 Carpenter Road Chester, NY 10918 Phone: 800-624-9600 www.repro-med.com
RITA Medical Systems (Formerly HMP-Horizon Medical Products)	One Horizon Way PO Box 627 Manchester, GA 31816 Phone: 706-846-3126 www.hmpvascular.com
Smiths Medical (Formerly Deltec)	1265 Grey Fox Road St. Paul, MN 55112 Phone: 651-633-2556 www.smiths-medical.com
Vygon Corporation	2495 General Armistead Avenue Norristown, PA 19403 Phone: 800-544-4907 www.vygonusa.com

CHAPTER 7

Quality Assurance

Providers of outpatient parenteral antimicrobial therapy (OPAT) must maintain a certain level of risk management, preferably under the umbrella of a broad quality assurance program. The concept of providing hospital-quality care in outpatient facilities and in the home setting is relatively new and accompanied by some risk. Although the technology that makes OPAT possible is not always tried and proven, increasing pressures to avoid or reduce hospitalization continue to stimulate its growth. Little is known, however, about how far outpatient care can reasonably be expanded and what its limits should be.

Not every patient who needs intravenous (IV) medication can or should be treated in an outpatient setting. The outcomes measures to test OPAT's safety and quality are in the early stage of development, and the monitoring systems are not yet firmly in place. This is not surprising, since even conventional medicine still lacks good tools to justify the current "standards of practice." The Infectious Diseases Society of America's (IDSA's) 2004 Practice Guidelines for Outpatient Parenteral Antimicrobial Therapy updates those published in 1997, with particular emphasis on quality measures and outcomes indicators.[1] The OPAT Outcomes Registry is a national database which helps compare the performance of individual programs with that of an aggregate of 30-plus centers representing more than 14,000 patients.[1-3] Outpatient parenteral antimicrobial therapy centers collect data on patient outcomes and can monitor their own clinical performances over time. Performance data are particularly useful in the absence of published outcomes standards for infections treated with OPAT.

Quality assurance in health care is an evolving concept. The overall quality of care in the outpatient setting should be comparable to that required in the hospital, although clearly many of the risks are different. We need to know more about the nature and importance of those risks. Of some concern is the recent report of complications of OPAT from a survey of infectious diseases specialists.[4]

Protocols and guidelines that have been developed by individual OPAT programs and home infusion companies vary greatly and may be proprietary.[5] Standardization is hindered by the rapid changes taking place in the industry in response to advances in technology as well as changing financial incentives (see Chapter 8). Quality assurance activities required or recommended by accrediting and licensing bodies have generally been focused on compliance with patient care processes and procedures rather than actual clinical outcomes as indicators of quality.

■ *OPAT Accreditation*

In the rush to provide some assurance of quality when contracting under managed care limitations, many third-party payers currently require that eligible OPAT programs have some kind of formal accreditation. During the past decade, the Joint Commission on Accreditation of Healthcare Organizations (JCAHO) has expanded its certification process to include outpatient and home care settings.[6]

The JCAHO home care accreditation program is second in size only to its hospital program. Accreditation is also available for mental health care, long-term health care, and ambulatory health care,[7] under which an accreditation process for ambulatory infusion centers was initiated in January 1995. Thus, physicians' office-based infusion centers are now eligible for JCAHO accreditation. (Infections Limited in Tacoma, Washington, was the first such center to be accredited.) In 1997, long-term care pharmacies, which provide infusion and other drug therapy to long-term care facilities, were included for JCAHO accreditation.[8] Organizations interested in applying for JCAHO accreditation may wish to access the JCAHO Website (www.jcaho.org) for information regarding accreditation requirements.

Most of the larger home infusion pharmacy provider organizations have earned JCAHO accreditation. Other providers have been accredited through the Community Health Accreditation Program (CHAP, www.chapinc.org), and some have the imprimatur of both.

A third agency, the Accreditation Association for Ambulatory Health Care (AAAHC, www.aaahc.org), surveys intermediate-provider components of managed care organizations, such as surgical centers and multispecialty group practices.[9] This organization also accredits college and university health centers, employee health programs, and infusion centers.

The AAAHC and JCAHO have signed a cooperative accreditation agreement allowing AAAHC accreditation to fulfill JCAHO standards for ambulatory care organizations in certain situations. For the purposes of this agreement, ambulatory care organizations include ambulatory surgery centers, endoscopy centers, office-based surgery sites, and medical group practices, as long as the organization is not part of a hospital's Medicare provider number.

The accreditation survey process is costly, with fees based on a provider's gross annual revenue (e.g., CHAP) or a base fee plus a variable amount calculated on patient volume and number of sites (e.g., JCAHO). The incentives to pursue accreditation are great, however. The majority of health insurance plans and managed care organizations requires it, and once accredited, agencies can receive "deemed status," which allows them to be reimbursed by Medicare and Medicaid without undergoing a separate certification process.

The JCAHO's focus changed in 1995 to emphasize actual performance (not simply the capacity to perform), as well as performance standards focused on quality improvement. Thus, indicators, defined as quantitative outcomes or process measures related to performance, have now become an integral part of the organization's accreditation process.

■ *Indicators of OPAT Quality*

A number of professional organizations have developed indicators of quality care that may eventually be incorporated into quality assurance standards specifically designed for OPAT. For example, the American Medical Association's (AMA's) Council on Scientific Affairs Report 9, *On-site Physician Home Health Care*,[10] a 2005 update of the AMA's *Physician Guide to Home Health Care*, addresses such general issues as physician education for home care, the communication revolution in home care, the new "electronic black bag" of miniaturized diagnostic technology and drug delivery devices, barriers to physician involvement, and conflicting regulatory and legal requirements. Antibiotic therapy is not specifically discussed, however.

The American Society of Health-System Pharmacists has written guidelines that define the role of the pharmacist in providing pharmaceutical care to patients in the home or alternate-site setting.[11]

The Infusion Nurses Society has published standards of practice for insertion, care, and maintenance of vascular access devices but has not adapted them to the outpatient setting.[12]

The Centers for Disease Control and Prevention has promulgated guidelines for "practitioners who insert catheters and for persons responsible for surveillance and control of infections in hospital, outpatient, and home health care settings."[13]

The U.S. Occupational Safety and Health Administration published a *Model Exposure Control Plan for Home Care: A Guide for Hospice/Home Care Agencies on Bloodborne Pathogen Standards* in 1994 but has released little else on home health care since.[14]

The Food and Drug Administration has a standing *MedWatch System* (http://fda.gov/medwatch/index.html) to track problems and adverse events associated with medications and medical devices, such as infusion pumps.

The IDSA's recently published guidelines include the basic criteria for an outpatient program, clinical monitoring of patients, and the qualifications of a program medical director.[1]

■ *Monitoring Outcomes*

As OPAT grows, objective measurements of its value must be developed. To accomplish this, providers must agree on criteria by which to measure program quality based on practical clinical outcome indicators. Ongoing monitoring of outcomes offers the additional advantage of identifying the comparative value of different therapeutic approaches. Today, more than ever, physicians must know more about the relative value of almost any therapy to justify it under the pressures of managed care. When is it appropriate to send a patient home with IV therapy? What is the best dosing regimen? When can oral antibiotics be used instead?

The measurement of outcomes by an OPAT program is a part of the continuous performance improvement process through which health care providers attempt to improve and ensure quality of their care and services. Accrediting bodies require outcomes measurements as a part of their certification process but do not specify the parameters or indicators to use. Therefore OPAT centers should have an active performance improvement program that can track clinical and program outcomes.

Tools with which to judge the quality of OPAT programs objectively were developed in the OPAT Outcomes Registry, which provided information about the most commonly treated infections (Figure 7.1), the pathogens found, and the primary antibiotics used, as well as outcomes indicators for patients treated with OPAT (Table 7.1).[1] Table 7.2 shows the outcomes of 7892 cases and 10,844 courses of antibiotic therapy provided from 1997 to 2001 in the United States.[2]

An International OPAT Outcomes Registry based on the US project includes data from the United Kingdom, Italy, and Canada. Over the 3 years from 1998 to 2001, 1141 cases have been entered from those

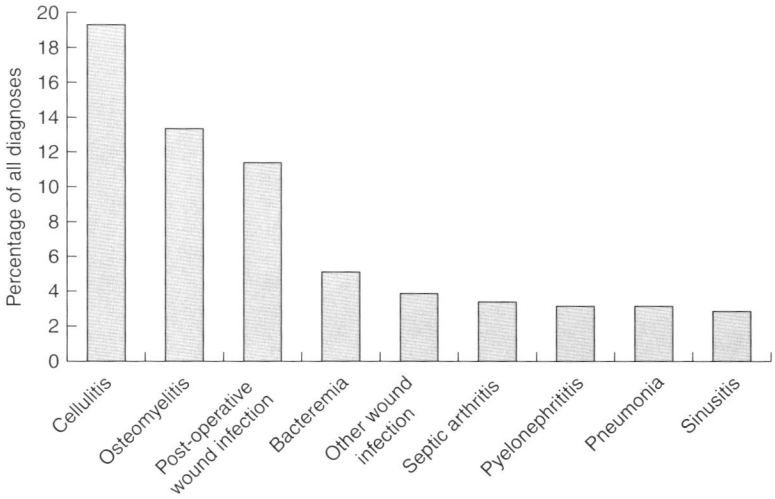

Figure 7.1. *Top 10 infections treated in the OPAT Outcomes Registry of 24 sites in the United States from 1997 to 2000. (Reprinted from Nathwani and Tice,[2] with permission.)*

Table 7.1.   Outcome Measures for Outpatient Parenteral Antimicrobial Therapy (OPAT)

1. Clinical status (as reported by responsible physcan)
   A. Improved
   B. Clinical failure
   C. No change

2. Bacterial infection status (if a pathogen was identified and repeat culture was done)
   A. Culture negative for pathogen
   B. Persistent pathogen
   C. New pathogen

3. Program outcome (i.e., end of therapy)
   A. Therapy completed as planned
   B. Therapy not completed because of patient's death, noncompliance with therapy, complication, patient's preference, hospitalization (give reason), or other

4. Antibiotic use (i.e., end of treatment course)
   A. Course completed as planned
   B. Course not completed because of adverse drug reaction (note type), resistant organism, persistent organism, patient's preference, clinical failure

5. Vascular access complications such as phlebitis, infection, thrombosis, infiltration, or becoming dislodged

6. Additional outcome measurements
   A. Patient returned to work or school during OPAT (if applicable)
   B. Did outcome meet physician expectations?
   C. Survival status (patient alive, died of infection, died of other causes, lost to follow-up, or status unknown)

Reprinted from Tice et al.,[1] with permission

countries.[2] These data can be used by OPAT organizations to compare their outcomes with those from their own countries or from the entire registry database.

An OPAT Outcomes Registry can also be used by local OPAT programs to evaluate and track their services. For example, it can be adapted to provide information on issues such as economics and patient satisfaction. The introduction of such quality indicators for evaluating one local practice proved valuable in terms of both quality improvement and service development (Table 7.3.)

Table 7.2. Outcomes Measures From the United States OPAT Outcomes Registry Based on 7892 Cases and 10,844 Courses of Antibiotic Therapy Provided From 1997 to 2001

Clinical outcomes [No.(%)]		
Improved	7189	(96.6)
Failed	92	(1.2)
No change	153	(2)
Bacterial outcomes [No.(%)]		
No culture	6614	(88.8)
Culture negative	666	(8.9)
Persistent pathogen	109	(1.5)
New pathogen	60	(0.8)
Program outcomes [No.(%)]		
Completed	7096	(92.2)
Ended early	323	(4.1)
Hospitalized	275	(3.5)
Died	39	(0.5)
Antibiotic outcomes [No.(%)]		
Completed	8715	(82.1)
Adverse event	492	(4.6)
Clinical failure	78	(0.7)
Resistant organism	44	(0.4)
Adverse events (*n* = 593)		
Rash	34	
Nausea/vomiting	12.8	
Fever	11.4	
Nephrotoxicity	7	

Reprinted from Nathwani and Tice,[2] with permission.

Patient safety and health care–related infections are of particular concern with OPAT.[15] The home environment is rarely constructed for safety; hence, application of hospital infection control policies may not be appropriate. Fortunately, the risk of infection related to home care appears to be much less than that related to hospitalization; patients' chances of acquiring antimicrobial-resistant organisms from the home environment seem to be much lower.[16]

Table 7.3. Quality Indicators for Infections Treated with Intravenous Antibiotics in the Outpatient and Home Setting Between April 1998 and August 2001 in Tayside, Scotland, United Kingdom

Infections treated (%)[a]	
Skin/soft tissue infections	54.5
Osteomyelitis/septic arthritis	22.2
Bacterial endocarditis	3.7
Others	19.6
Clinical outcomes (%)	
Cure	97.2
No change	1.8
Worse	1
Adverse drug reactions	2.4
Unscheduled re-admission	3
PICC[b] complications	1
Microbiological outcomes (%)	
Positive culture pre-treatment	20
Positive culture post-treatment	0
Economic outcome	
Number of patients treated	470
Total number of inpatient bed days saved	6,693
Additional daily cost of OPAT drugs per person	<6
Patient satisfaction (%)	
Treatment met or exceeded expectations	98.5
Preferred service to inpatient treatment	96.5
Would choose this form of treatment again	96.5

[a]These include meningitis, complicated urinary tract infections. MRSA wound infections and bacteremia, chest infections, cutancous leishmaniasis, etc.
[b]PICC, peripherally inserted central catheter.
Reprinted from Nathwani and Tice,[2] with permission.

In May 2004, the Emerging Infections Network (EIN) of the IDSA sent a survey to its 848 North American members—all infectious disease consultants (IDCs)—regarding the delivery of OPAT in their practice settings, their involvement in the process, and their observations about its use and safety.[4] A total of 452 (53%) members responded with relevant data. They collectively had followed more than 13,000 OPAT patients during the previous year, treating over 90% at home, using peripherally inserted central venous catheters for 86%. They used a variety of infusion devices.

During that year, however, more than 60% of EIN members collectively encountered approximately 1943 infectious and noninfectious complications (Figure 7.2).

The investigators concluded that most hospitals in North America have OPAT services, and IDCs frequently participate in the management and follow-up of these patients. The magnitude of OPAT operations and the frequency of complications suggest that additional investigation of this practice is warranted to improve the quality and safety of OPAT services.

The need for quality measures and performance indicators will only increase as medical care shifts out of the hospital and back into the community. Hospitals have evolved valuable mechanisms to improve patient care and safety under the watchful care of omnipresent medical staff and remarkable resources. Unfortunately, the cost of hospital care may no longer be justifiable. Patients, even those with serious infections, are increasingly being discharged early or not admitted at all. A safety net of providers and systems learned

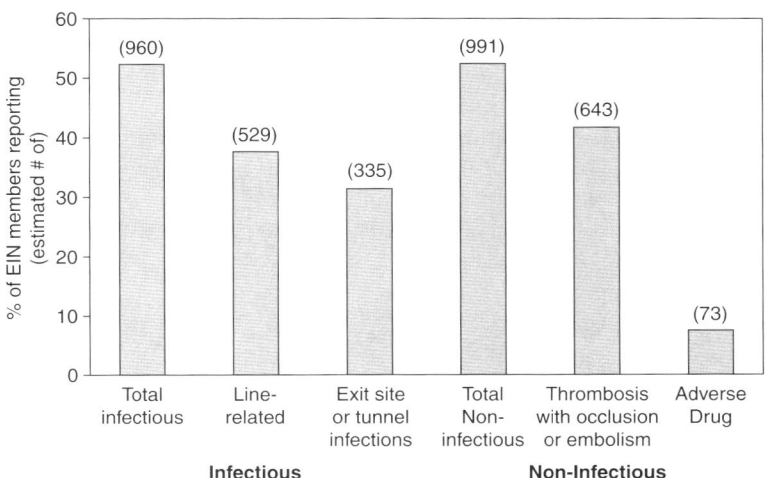

Figure 7.2. *Complications of OPAT in 2003. (Reprinted from Strausbaugh and Tice,[4] with permission.)*

Table 7.4.   Criteria for Evaluation and Selection of an OPAT Provider

1. Medical director or advisor knowledgeable in infectious diseases and OPAT
2. Outlined roles of prescribing physician, medical director, nurse, and pharmacist
3. Standards for nurse, pharmacist, physician, and other patient care personnel regarding training, experience, and licensure
4. Accreditation or certification (e.g., JCAHO)
5. Experience providing OPAT
6. Policies regarding
   - Frequency of physician and nurse clinical assessments
   - Staffing and on-call policies
   - Frequency of reports to physicians
7. Reporting of laboratory results to physicians within 24 hours
8. Willingness to share local quality assurance and outcomes information
9. Willingness to share charge information regarding individual patients

From 1996 IDSA Task Force on HOPAT Standards, with permission.

---

from hospital experience needs to be established in order to ensure effective therapy with minimal risks.

■ Selecting an OPAT Program

Factors to be considered by physicians in selecting an OPAT provider agency are outlined in Table 7.4. Although not complete, the outline may provide referring physicians with a useful checklist of the basic elements required of any program that provides IV infusion therapy. The referring physician must always keep in mind, however, that he or she remains responsible for the referred patient's care regardless of who actually administers it. The checklist also may be helpful in making comparisons among available programs.

References

1. Tice AD, Rehm SJ, Dalovisio JR, et al. Practice guidelines for outpatient parenteral antimicrobial therapy. IDSA guidelines. *Clin Infect Dis.* 2004;38:1651–1672.
2. Nathwani D, Tice A. Ambulatory antimicrobial use: the value of an outcomes registry. *J Antimicrob Chemother.* 2002;49:149–154.
3. The OPAT Outcomes Registry. Available at: www.opat.com. Accessed June 9, 2005.
4. Strausbaugh LJ, Tice AD, Martinelli OJP, et al. Experience of infectious diseases consultants with outpatient parenteral antimicrobial therapy: results of an emerging infections network service. Poster presented at: 15th Annual Scientific Meeting of the Society for Healthcare Epidemiology of America (SHEA); April 9–12, 2005; Los Angeles, CA.

5. Balinsky W, Mollin A. Home drug infusion therapy. A literature update. *Int J Technol Assess Health Care*. 1998;14:535–543.

6. *2004-2005 Comprehensive Accreditation Manual for Home Care (CAMHC)*. Oakbrook Terrace, IL: Joint Commission on Accreditation of Healthcare Organizations.

7. *2005-2006 Comprehensive Accreditation Manual for Ambulatory Care (CAMAC)*. Oakbrook Terrace, IL: Joint Commission on Accreditation of Healthcare Organizations.

8. *2004–2005 Standards for Dispensing Pharmacy, Clinical/Consultant Pharmacist, Long Term Care Pharmacy, and Freestanding Ambulatory Infusion Services*. Oakbrook Terrace, IL: Joint Commission on Accreditation of Healthcare Organizations.

9. *2005 Accreditation Handbook for Ambulatory Health Care*. Skokie, IL: Accreditation Association for Ambulatory Health Care.

10. Council on Scientific Affairs Report 9. *On-site Physician Home Health Care*. Chicago, IL: American Medical Association; 2005.

11. American Society of Health-System Pharmacists. ASHP guidelines on the pharmacist's role in home care. *Am J Health Syst Pharm*. 2000;57:1252–1257.

12. Infusion Nurses Society. Infusion nursing standards of practice. *J Intraven Nurs*. 2002;23(suppl 6):S1–S88.

13. O'Grady NP, Alexander M, Dellinger EP, et al. Guidelines for the prevention of intravascular catheter-related infections. *MMWR Recomm Rep*. 2002;51(RR-10):1–29.

14. Occupational Safety and Health Administration. *Model Exposure Control Plan for Home Care: A Guide for Hospice/Home Agencies on Bloodborne Pathogen Standards*. Washington, DC: U.S. Government Printing Office; 1994.

15. Embry FC, Chinnes I.F. Draft definitions for surveillance of infections in home health care. *Am J Infect Control*. 2000;28:449-453.

16. Tice AD, Barrett T. Home health care. In: Abrutyn E, Goldmann DA, Scheckler WE, eds. Saunders *Infection Control Reference Service. The Experts' Guide to the Guidelines*. 2nd ed. Philadelphia, PA: WB Saunders; 2001.

CHAPTER 8

Reimbursement

The stance taken by third-party payers regarding reimbursement for outpatient parenteral antimicrobial therapy (OPAT) has changed dramatically over the years. Originally, payers were reluctant to approve OPAT because of its novelty and concerns about its safety. Once they understood its value and its potential savings compared with the usual $1,000 per day spent in the hospital, this attitude changed. At first, fees for outpatient care were considerably higher than they are today, and profit margins for care providers were generous but still low relative to those submitted by hospitals.

With the increased acceptance of outpatient care by providers and the public, however, payers now *expect* beneficiaries to be treated as outpatients. Many insurance companies no longer consider intravenous (IV) antibiotic therapy a criterion for hospitalization, even if two drugs are needed. The patient may simply be told he or she will have to pay the hospital costs or be shuffled off to an extended care facility to complete the course of therapy. A competitive environment has often led to dramatic reductions in OPAT charges—and probably to quality of care as well.

Furthermore, many insurance regulators and rate setters perceive home care as two separate clinical categories, service providers and medical products, rather than as an inseparable combination of both. The result is often a confusion of deductibles and requirements for reimbursement.

Table 8.1.   Reimbursement for Outpatient IV Antimicrobial Therapy

Payer	Coverage Service	Reimbursement	Codes
Medicare	Drugs	EAC or AWP	J-Code[a]
	DME, supplies, services	Payment for specific drugs and supplies under DME benefit billed to the DME Reimbursement Code or for drugs and procedures provided by the physician in his or her office.	HCPCS[b] CPT[c]
Commercial insurance (e.g., Blue Cross/ Blue Shield)	Drugs	AWP	J-Code, NDC
	DME, supplies, services	Payment varies by contract, usually 80% to 100% of covered charges may be per diem.	HCPCS, CPT
Medicaid (may require prior approval)	Drugs	AWP varies by state	J-Code, NDC
	DME, supplies, services	Varies by state	HCPCS, CPT

[a]Medicare, Medicaid, and most other payers use the Health Care Financing Administration common procedure coding system (HCPCS) for drugs—"J-Codes."
[b]Health care common procedure coding system (equipment and drugs).
[c]AMA current procedural terminology (services).
Abbreviations: AWP, average wholesale price; DME, durable medical equipment; EAC, estimated acquisition cost; NDC, national drug code.
From Balinsky[3] with permission.

Adapted from Balinsky WI. Home IV drug therapy reimbursement. In Conners RB, Winters RW, eds. *Home Infusion: Current Status and Figure Trends*. Chicago, IL. American Hospital Publishing, 1995.

This chapter is an attempt to clarify the various reimbursement policies for OPAT of the major third-party payers: Medicare, commercial insurers, and Medicaid (Table 8.1). Because most OPAT is delivered in patients' homes, and the least standardized and most bewildering reimbursement policies are those pertaining to home care, that will be the predominant focus.

The complexities of OPAT reimbursement require a clear understanding of what payers will pay and to whom. Contracts are in order for private payers, and a thorough and up-to-date knowledge of state and federal policies is necessary before a program is initiated and, once started, close attention to periodic policy modifications is required. Also crucial to a program's success is the institution of a rigid policy to require prior authorization for OPAT from private payers—with the date, time, and person involved—and preferably a fax to confirm. Assuming payment in a timely manner has been the downfall of many OPAT programs, particularly with the high cost of some products, such as immune globulin and immune modulators.

■ *Medicare*

Medicare is a federal health insurance program primarily for people older than 65 years, for certain disbled persons, and for anyone with permanent kidney failure.

Because Medicare does not pay money directly to health care providers but has different fiscal intermediaries and carriers, policies may be interpreted differently in different locales. However, the basic facts regarding eligibility and coverage can be useful. The program has two mechanisms for reimbursement, Part A and Part B.[1,2] Neither will guarantee or give preauthorization for payment, although coverage is carefully outlined by the Centers for Medicare & Medicaid Services (CMS) as well as local intermediaries. As of 2006, a Medicare Part D benefit will cover prescription drugs for qualified beneficiaries with a number of limitations and criteria yet to be defined.[3]

Medicare Part A

Part A covers hospital services, limited services at a skilled nursing facility, some home care services, and hospice services. Premiums, deductibles, and coinsurance payments may be required.

To meet home care requirements, patients must be confined at home and require intermittent (at least once every 60 days but not daily for longer than a short time period) and skilled care as determined by a physician. In other words, continuous service and custodial care are excluded. Skilled service is that provided by a skilled nurse, physical therapist, or speech therapist. Once eligible for these services, a patient also may take advantage of occupational therapy, medical social services, and a home health aide.

Also included with skilled service are some medical equipment and supplies. Drugs are not included, nor are home infusion services, although skilled nursing visits to support such services may be reimbursed under specific circumstances. For Medicare patients who require infusion therapy, early discharge programs, some of which are managed by physicians, may be covered by the hospital.[4]

Medicare Part B

Part B expands Part A to include physician services, ambulance transportation, prosthetic devices, independent laboratory tests, and a limited number of drugs and biological agents administered in outpatient clinics. Because it includes the durable medical equipment (DME) portion of reimbursement, Part B covers selected home IV drug therapy, including only 4 antimicrobials (acyclovir, ganciclovir, amphotericin, foscarnet), based on the need for an infusion pump (if durable and reusable).

Such pumps must be external and can be either portable or stationary. Neither elastomeric devices (which are disposable, single-use systems) nor implantable pumps are covered. Furthermore, external pumps are covered only when a prolonged infusion (at least 8 hours) is necessary or when a controlled rate is needed to avoid toxicity and an alternative method (such as a drip infusion or an elastomeric infusion pump) is not acceptable. When this benefit applies, the pump itself is covered as well as the drug and infusion supplies. The infusion may be self-administered but the drug must be supplied by a registered DME provider. Physicians can be DME providers. The alternative for Medicare patients who need drugs not covered under the DME provisions and/or are unable to pay for OPAT privately are to stay in the hospital, go to a skilled nursing care facility, or receive OPAT through a hospital outpatient program or physician office-based program.

Medicare will pay for outpatient infusion of drugs when the drug is administered by a physician directly or by employees of a physician under his or her direct supervision. Thus, the physician must be present or immediately at hand when the patient is receiving care, whether in the office or home. Payment may be denied if a physician is not present, even if a nurse administers IV antibiotics following a physician's orders. Some carriers have recently allowed nurse practitioners or physician assistants to replace physicians in this supervisory role.

Physician "care plan oversight" of home health patients only applies to home infusion patients when they require comprehensive management through a certified home health agency.[5,6] With proper documentation, physicians should be able to submit many claims for these services to Medicare patients.

When covered, services and supplies are reimbursed at 80% of the published Medicare allowable fee. Patients should be aware of the

20% co-payment which, in some cases, may be prohibitive. Supplemental (Medi-Gap) insurance carriers will pay the 20% co-pay of anything covered by Medicare. Payment for the drug is currently published quarterly and is based on the Average Sales Price (ASP) plus 6%, methodology established in 2005 under direction from Congress.[7]

Any OPAT program that is willing and able to provide care for Medicare patients will need to keep up with the programs' changing regulations and reimbursement plans.

■ *Medicaid*

Sponsored by both federal and state governments, Medicaid is actually 50 different, state-run, health insurance programs. Eligible groups are people who require financial aid, usually recipients of public assistance; medically needy people who are blind or disabled; and people younger than age 21 years and older than age 65 years whose family caretaker is incapacitated or has a catastrophic illness. In general, Medicaid coverage is broader and more generous than Medicare.

Although most prescription and some nonprescription drugs are covered, IV antibiotics require prior approval. Some Medicaid programs have added multidisciplinary case-management services that use outpatient and home care as a cost-efficient way of providing quality care.

Physicians who wish Medicaid patients to be treated at home should inquire about payment from the state department of social services, which handles all Medicaid issues. Typically, a physician or home health care agency that requests prior approval for reimbursement must submit a plan of care to Medicaid that details the medicines and other supplies that will be required. The agency or physician will bill Medicaid for the cost of visits and equipment; the dispensing pharmacy or physician will bill Medicaid directly for the cost of drugs.

Administration of drugs with an infusion pump is not a prerequisite for Medicaid coverage, as it is with Medicare. Reimbursement for the antimicrobial is usually based on the average acquisition cost determined via state databases or invoices.

State AIDS Drug Assistance Programs and compassionate use funds provided by many pharmaceutical companies may also be a source of reimbursement for OPAT for indigent or low-income patients.

■ *Commercial Insurers*

Most private insurance policies today have some provision for outpatient benefits, although some lower-priced policies cover catastrophic costs of hospitalization only, or they specifically exclude outpatient prescription drug coverage that may include parenteral medications. In some cases, it may be possible for a provider to negotiate coverage under these policies in lieu of hospitalization, but this requires direct contact with someone who has the authority to make such decisions. Some policies still cover all outpatient care at a lower percentage of billed charges than those of hospitalization, which can result in prohibitive costs for many patients.

Insurance companies may dictate which providers will be reimbursed for OPAT and/or require prior authorization for treatment. For example, OPAT charges may be covered at a lower percentage or not at all if the beneficiary does not use a "preferred provider" who has contracted with the payer. Or pre- and ongoing authorization by the primary care physician (as in an HMO) or insurance case manager may be required. In the absence of a contracted preferred provider, preauthorization may involve price negotiation.

It is essential that providers minimize their financial risk, as well as that of their patients, by gathering all the necessary information regarding coverage before initiating OPAT. The advent of managed care has led to an increase in the number of insurance companies that require authorization and management of OPAT by a case manager employed by the company itself. Providers will find a positive working relationship with these managers to be essential.

■ *Billing*

Insurance plans also have varying policies regarding how charges are billed. Claim forms, codes, and required documentation may vary widely. The Health Insurance Portability and Accountability Act of 1996 (HIPAA) regulations call for standardization by the industry, which, hopefully, can be achieved in the near future.[8]

Itemized Billing

Many plans require itemized billing of charges associated with OPAT. These payers list every unit of drug and supply, often marked up to include fixed overhead costs, as well as codes for any procedures or services related to the therapy.

Charges may be paid in full or, as is more likely, at the payer's "usual and customary" rate. Itemized billing cannot capture the cognitive services often involved in providing OPAT, which led to the development of per diem billing.

Per Diem Billing

An increasingly common method for billing OPAT products and services is the set charge for each day a patient is on therapy. The per diem fee, which usually is separate from the charges for antibiotics, covers all administration supplies, nursing care, pharmaceutical services, cognitive services, and overhead for the 24 hours a provider must be on call for a patient receiving infusion therapy.

This type of reimbursement allows providers greater flexibility and rewards cost-efficient delivery of services, and provides the payer with a predictable estimated cost for the therapy, regardless of unforeseen circumstances. Some negotiated contracts for per diem reimbursement allow for the additional care required by more severely ill patients by including a fixed number of nursing visits in the fee and separate billing for authorized visits beyond that number. Some policies also build in gradations to allow for multiple or more complex therapies or for specialized care, such as that required by patients with AIDS.

■ *Risk Sharing*

There are to date minimal experience and data to support providers in negotiating reasonable risk-sharing arrangements. In most markets where capitation is the growing mechanism for reimbursement, OPAT is often "carved out" or excluded from the services under capitation, and a per diem fee is set for contracted OPAT providers. Some larger companies and specialist physicians have entered into agreements whereby OPAT is either included in the total per member per month (PMPM) reimbursement for all care, or home care (including home infusion) or infusion therapy has its own PMPM reimbursement.[9]

Such arrangements give providers, physicians in particular, a great deal of flexibility in treatment and help streamline program administration in terms of billing and collections. However, capitation agreements should be entered into with caution, given the high costs involved in OPAT delivery, due primarily to requirements for a large drug inventory and the employment of specialized personnel. Providers who are able to collect meaningful data regarding the patient population they serve and the cost of providing OPAT are in the best position to consider this kind of risk-sharing agreement.

Table 8.2. Major Reimbursement Coding Systems

Service	Coding System	
Diagnosis	ICD-9	International Classification of Diseases, Ninth Revision
Office visit	CPT	Current Procedural Terminology
	E&M	Evaluation and Management
Drug/product	HCPCS	Health Care Common Procedure Coding System (e.g., J-Code)
	NDC	National Drug Code
Procedure	CPT	Current Procedural Terminology

■ Coding

No discussion of reimbursement is complete without mention of coding systems used for computer identification of the diagnosis, the medical service, place of service, and the drug administered. If codes are missing or incorrect or do not match, claims are processed manually, thus increasing the chances of their being delayed, denied, or paid incorrectly. The major reimbursement coding systems are listed in Table 8.2.[10]

Even though not all payers cover all three charges for OPAT (the visit, the procedure, and the medication) under all circumstances, a good rule of thumb when submitting claims is to include all three, as well as applicable codes for the visit, diagnosis, procedure, and medication.

Because of the complexity of reimbursement, many pharmaceutical companies offer assistance and advice about billing for their products. This information can be accessed through their Websites and their local sales force.

References

1. U.S. Congress, Office of Technology Assessment. *Home Drug Infusion Therapy Under Medicare.* Chapter OTA-H-509. Washington, DC: U.S. Government Printing Office; May 1992.

2. Tice AD, Hoaglund PA, Nolet B, et al. Cost perspectives for outpatient intravenous antimicrobial therapy. *Pharmacotherapy.* 2002;22(Suppl):63S–70S.

3. Centers for Medicare & Medicaid Services. Medicare fee-for-service part B drugs. Available at: www.cms.hhs.gov/providers/drugs. Accessed August 11, 2005.

4. Hindes R, Winkler C, Kane P, et al. Outpatient intravenous antibiotic therapy in Medicare patients: cost savings analysis. *Infect Dis Clin Pract.* 1995;4:211–217.

5. Friend A, ed. *The Complete Guide to Medicare Physician Payment for Home Health and Hospice Care Plan Oversight.* Rockville, MD: United Communications Group; 2004.

6. Infectious Diseases Society of America. Practice Management Resources and Tools. Available at: www.idsociety.org. Accessed August 13, 2005.

7. Centers for Medicare & Medicaid Services. Medicare prescription drug coverage. "It's all coming together." Available at: www.cms.hhs.gov. Accessed August 11, 2005.

8. Centers for Medicare & Medicaid Services. The Health Insurance Portability and Accountability Act of 1996 (HIPAA). Available at: www.cms.hhs.gov/hipaa. Accessed August 12, 2005.

9. Tice AD, Slama TG, Berman S, et al. Managed care and the infectious diseases specialist. *Clin Infect Dis.* 1996;23:341–368.

10. Tierce JC. Reimbursement. *Hosp Pract.* 1993;28(suppl 1):44–51.

CHAPTER 9

Legal Issues

Although outpatient parenteral antimicrobial therapy (OPAT) is relatively new and not yet well defined in terms of ethics, regulations, and the law, several issues of concern have already been identified. First, the medical risks associated with the outpatient setting are different from those in the hospital. Patients and their families should be informed of these risks and know their own responsibilities in regard to them.

Patients cannot be as closely monitored at home, for example, and will not have the same ready access to a physician or nurse. They must take responsibility for monitoring their own symptoms as well as for identifying and reporting problems. They must comply with the scheduling and travel requirements of the delivery model agreed upon with the referring physician and the home infusion team. It is common practice for patients to sign a document that indicates they have been informed of the potential risks and problems involved with outpatient therapy and that they have had an opportunity to discuss them in full with a physician. Legally, such forms may deter lawsuits and may be helpful in defense, but they do not ensure victory in the courtroom. The Health Insurance Portability and Accountability Act of 1996 (HIPAA) regulations are now a required part of any outpatient treatment facility and an indication of the concerns about patient confidentiality as well as electronic information management.[1]

Patients may have to make choices among intravenous (IV) therapy providers. The prescribing physician may be helpful in selecting the provider, based on his or her knowledge of the chosen provider's quality of service as well as his or her ability to work with that provider. Also important is the prescribing physician's willingness to take responsibility for the care provided. Patients should be informed of the mechanism for reporting complaints, both within and outside the provider organization. And they should be given information regarding the ownership of the provider organization, particularly, if the referring physician is an owner on any level.

Finally, Medicare beneficiaries are protected by a law that requires all providers to inform them of uncovered services to be rendered, as well as a written estimate of any financial responsibility incurred, before beginning treatment.[2]

■ Antitrust Law

Federal antitrust policies, generally developed through court decisions rather than mandated by legislation, have been designed to protect consumers from high prices, price fixing, and limitation of choice among goods or services.[3,4] Physicians and other health care providers cannot form organizations simply to reduce competition or fix prices for medical services. Specific guidelines define acceptable arrangements and situations in which exceptions may apply. In 1996, legislation widened the safety net for physician providers.[3,4] However, any provider considering participation in joint ventures, networks, or integrated delivery systems should consult a qualified antitrust law specialist in order to minimize the risk of running afoul of these complex regulations.

■ Professional Liability

Much of OPAT's growth has resulted from the efforts of pharmacists, nurses, and business entrepreneurs. Physicians have lagged behind in their interest and involvement in outpatient and home therapy, in part, because of the lack of reimbursement for patient care services in this setting. Furthermore, the concept of managing sicker patients in a setting without continuous hands-on assessment and intervention is difficult for many physicians to embrace. Many infectious diseases specialists do not even have an office in which to see patients for follow-up.

Thus, in many programs a nurse or pharmacist is primarily responsible for patient care, with a physician merely signing forms and providing little actual direction. Physicians often may not even be involved in the choice of home care provider or in supervision of the quality of care provided their patients. Nevertheless, although nurses and pharmacists carry a certain degree of risk in terms of professional liability, physicians should be aware that they remain responsible and liable for the quality of care delivered to patients, even if they do not deliver it personally.

The classic model of the physician as "captain of the ship" has been tested repeatedly and proven in court. That leaves the ultimate responsibility for patient care to the physician who orders the treatment, selects the OPAT provider(s), and monitors the patient during the course of therapy.

Malpractice litigation related to outpatient and home care is rising. Lawsuits related to OPAT specifically are hard to track but seem to be increasing. OPAT problems may be less susceptible to lawsuits because of greater patient participation in the therapy provided, as well as general satisfaction with the benefits of the outpatient setting. However, in a recent survey of infectious diseases specialists, 4% of respondents reported having been sued in the past with respect to an OPAT matter.[5] As more and sicker patients are cared for in, or are discharged to, outpatient settings, an increase in recorded case law may be seen. So far the problems seem to focus around inadequate availability of and follow-up by physicians and aminoglycoside toxicity.

■ *Physician Conflict of Interest and Self-Referral*

Monetary incentives for physicians that may interfere with their clinical judgment and therapeutic parsimony are generally considered unethical and illegal. If, for example, physicians own or have a financial interest in an outpatient care provider organization, concern has arisen that they will overprescribe services, including home infusion therapy.[6]

On the other hand, if physicians are not involved in overseeing the quality of the services provided, patients may be ill-served and programs may suffer as a result. It is becoming more and more difficult to get physicians to spend the time, work, and energy required for such involvement, however, despite the fact that they are ultimately responsible for patient outcomes. The situation is largely the result of poor, usually absent payment to physicians for their management of patients being cared for at home. There is little incentive for physicians to discharge patients when they are paid for daily hospital visits but for only two or three office visits a week despite similar risks and responsibilities.

In response to concern regarding overuse of services for patients on Medicare, U.S. Representative Fortney (Pete) Stark of California sponsored legislation that attempts to regulate and restrict physician ownership and other financial arrangements with some services to which they refer patients.[7] At this time, federal regulations apply only to Medicare and Medicaid beneficiaries, although some states have passed similar legislation that extends restrictions to patients whose health care is funded through private insurance plans.[8] The assumption is that any ownership interest in, or payments from, provider organizations are inducements to overuse their services, as well as a conflict of interest in terms of a physician's role as patient advocate and judge of quality of care.

■ *Options for Physician Involvement in OPAT*

Under current stringent laws, rules, and regulations, there are still four ways for a physician to participate in OPAT: (1) by providing care plan oversight services (see Chapter 8); (2) as paid medical director of a hospital-, pharmacy-, or home health care company–based program; (3) by providing the service as an extension of his or her medical practice; and (4) by becoming a member of a physician–network joint venture.

Consultation with a competent health care attorney who is familiar with both state and federal regulations is an important step before finalizing the structure of any ownership or compensation agreement related to OPAT. However, safe harbors and reasonable exemptions exist whereby physicians can provide OPAT services as an extension of their practices and remain in compliance with relevant regulations. A physician who provides actual management services related to all patients of an OPAT provider organization and is compensated at fair market value may continue the relationship even while referring some or all of his/her patients on OPAT to that entity.

A physician–network joint venture is defined by the Department of Justice and Federal Trade Commission as a physician-controlled organization in which members collectively agree on prices or other significant terms of competition and jointly market their services.[3–4,6] Policy statements by the Department of Justice and Federal Trade Commission describe how antitrust laws apply to such organizations and establish "safety zones," within which their conduct will not be challenged by the federal antitrust agencies. There are, however, significant antitrust risks associated with joint ventures. Qualified antitrust counseling should be sought by any physician considering participation in such a network.

■ *Licensure and Medications*

Most requirements for licensure of an OPAT program will be dictated by the state where care and services are provided. Some payers, including Medicare and Medicaid, may require specific licensure, certification, or accreditation in order to contract with a provider. It is best to contact the State Board of Licensing to determine the requirements for a particular model or setting in a given state.

In most states, two OPAT services require licensure, registration, or compliance with published standards. One is the provision of hands-on nursing care in a patient's home, for which a state home health agency license may be required. The other is preparation and dispensing of medications for patient self-administration at home. The administration of drugs on-site will usually fall under the licensure of the professional or the facility where the infusion occurs (e.g., a physician's office, a hospital outpatient department). However, once a drug is given to the patient to take home, the State Board of Pharmacy has full purview in dictating licensure required or regulations to guide practice. In some states—Texas and Virginia, for example—even a physician's office must include a licensed retail pharmacy in order to dispense medications. Other states require only that guidelines regarding preparation, labeling, and transport are followed. All questions about dispensing are best asked of your State Board of Pharmacy, which can be accessed through the National Association of Boards of Pharmacy (www.nabp.net).

As of January 1, 2006, a new set of federal regulations now govern all preparation of medications that will not be administered immediately. Commonly referred to as USP 797, these regulations were developed in response to a number of cases of contaminated solutions due, at least in part, to the methods and environment for compounding. For further information, see Chapter 10.

■ *The Future*

As managed care and global capitation become more common, issues of self-referral and conflict of interest will be more focused on concerns regarding underuse rather than overuse of services. In the managed care environment, nonphysicians usually set practice guidelines and parameters. A case in point is a 1986 court decision holding the physician responsible for the loss of a patient's leg from gangrene.[9] The patient had been discharged earlier than the doctor had advised due to pressures from an HMO. The court held the physician negligent because he did not more strenuously object to the discharge.

Medicine and the law seem inseparable. Although regulations and legislation have attempted to provide some degree of quality assurance in medicine, good intentions have often led to unexpected and unwanted outcomes, with intrusions into patient care that seem, at times, to be ridiculous. With the changes in both medical care delivery and financing, new relationships are under scrutiny. Allegations of overuse in the fee-for-service system are countered by those of underuse associated with managed care.

The combination of government and consumer interest in controlling costs and ensuring high-quality patient care will undoubtedly continue to foster additional legislative and regulatory initiatives.

It is important for anyone involved with medicine to be aware of the regulations as well as potential legal and ethical problems, which are being constructed and defined. To what extent they will benefit the quality of patient care and improve the use of available resources remains to be determined, especially in the outpatient setting.

References

1. Centers for Medicare & Medicaid Services. The Health Insurance Portability and Accountability Act of 1996 (HIPAA). Available at: www.cms.hhs.gov/hipaa. Accessed August 12, 2005.

2. OBRA 1989, Public Law 101–239, Stat 2106.

3. Johnson J. New antitrust policy offers big gains for doctor networks. *Am Med News.* 1996;39:1–43.

4. Physician-run health plans and antitrust. American College of Physicians. *Ann Intern Med.* 1996;125:59–65.

5. Strausbaugh LJ, Tice AD, Martinelli OP, et al. Experience of infectious diseases consultants with outpatient parenteral antimicrobial therapy: results of an emerging infections network service. Poster presented at: 15th Annual Scientific Meeting of the Society for Healthcare Epidemiology of America (SHEA); April 9–12, 2005; Los Angeles, CA.

6. Tice AD, Slama TG, Berman S, et al. Managed care and the infectious diseases specialist. *Clin Infect Dis* 1996;23:341–368.

7. Department of Health and Human Services. Medicare Program: Physicians' referrals to health care entities with which they have financial relationships. Phase II Federal Register: March 26, 2004;69(39):16053-16146. Phase I Federal Register: January 4, 2000;66(3):855–904.

8. California Assembly Bill No. 919. Physician Ownership and Referral Act.

9. Wickline v State of California, Court of Appeals 2nd Dist, Div 5 (July 30, 1986). 192 Cal App 3rd 1630. 239 Cal. Rptr. 810.

CHAPTER 10

The Infusion Suite

This chapter is concerned primarily with the actual physical components and major design elements of an infusion suite regardless of the setting. Not included here are pharmacy design, issues, and regulations, which will be highly individualized based on the size of the practice, the population served, and State Board of Pharmacy regulations governing medication preparation and dispensing. It is important to note, however, that as of January 1, 2006, new federal regulations developed by the *United States Pharmacopeia* (USP) went into effect in the United States.

These regulations, which will be enforced by the U.S. Food and Drug Administration and the Joint Commission on Accreditation of Healthcare Organizations (JCAHO), target the preparation of dispensed medications, with an exception for those used immediately (defined as use that begins within 1 hour and is completed within 12 hours of noncontaminated preparation). All other sterile preparations, including the puncture of proprietary bag and vial systems (e.g., ADD-Vantage® and Mini-Bag Plus®) must meet the requirements outlined. The regulations and proposals for revisions and updates can be accessed on the USP Website (www.usp.org)

■ The Basics

The basic elements of an intravenous (IV) therapy suite are shown in Figure 10.1. Although the arrangement of these components will depend on the configuration and size of the space available, the

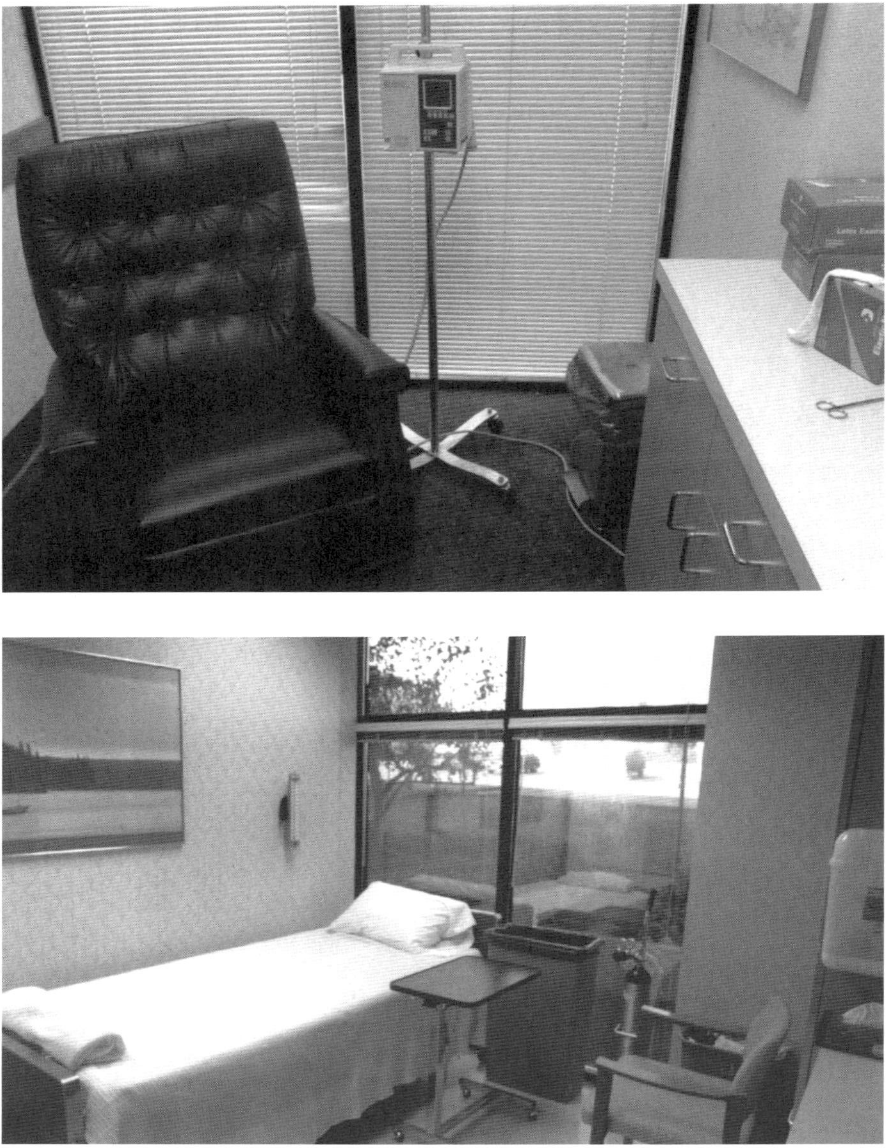

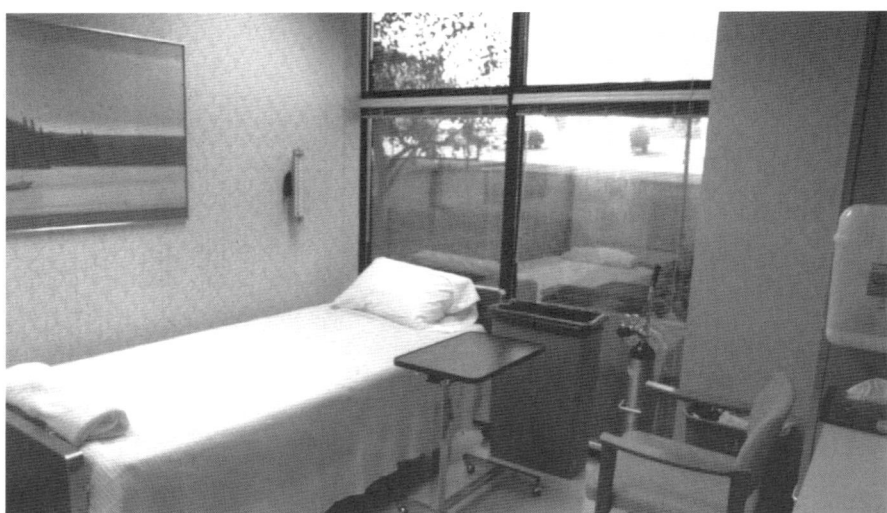

Figure 10.1   *Basic components of an outpatient intravenous therapy suite: comfortable bed or chair for the patient; chair for the physician, nurse, or a guest; good lighting, preferably natural light; infusion apparatus; sinks and countertops for cleanliness and work space; adequate space for staff or visitor; blinds or curtains for privacy.*

major clinical considerations should be efficiency, safety, work flow, and patient comfort and privacy. Needless to say, thought also should be given to the needs and comfort of the staff. Some questions that have bearing on spatial organization of any suite include

- Is there a need for the isolation of some patients?
- Should children have special accommodations?
- How should disruptive patients be accommodated?
- Will physicians be using the space for office visits and treatment of patients in addition to infusion therapy?
- Will special procedures, such as peripherally inserted central venous catheter (PICC) line insertion be performed in the room?

A number of basic components and general design features should be considered for all infusion suites regardless of size.

Lighting. Daylight is preferable for accurate assessment of patients' skin color and tissue perfusion. Alternative full-spectrum fluorescent lighting helps in both patient examination and in finding veins.

Temperature control. Ideally, separate ventilation and temperature control should be possible in each room to accommodate patient preferences and conditions. Ventilation systems are also important in controlling temperature as well as delivering fresh or purified air.

Visibility. All patient rooms should be visible from the nurses' station. If this is not possible, a visual or alarm call system may be helpful.

Privacy. All rooms should be equipped with doors or at least curtains between patients to allow privacy. A separate exit door may also be helpful for confidentiality.

Space. At least 4 feet of space on either side of the bed or recliner should be provided for nurses and physicians to care for patients, as well as for wheelchair access.

Cleanliness. All finish materials should be washable: washable paint or vinyl wall covering on walls; ceilings of either washable acoustic tile or gypsum wallboard with washable paint. Floors should be covered with linoleum, sheet goods, or washable carpet specifically designed to provide easy removal of blood and bodily fluids. Vertical blinds are preferable to horizontal blinds because they are easier to clean.

Durability. Wainscoting (about 4 feet high) is helpful since recliners and wheelchairs hitting against gypsum wallboard can cause significant damage. Although traditional wood wainscoting is generally more attractive, other materials, such as plastic laminate, are acceptable.

Sinks. If it is not possible to have a sink in every room, a centrally located sink and counter area can be used for staff and patient hand-washing, as well as initial training of patients in hand-washing technique. This area also may be used for cleaning equipment. A second sink at waist level can be useful for patients to "soak" their arms in hot water in order to facilitate venipuncture. Alcohol-based hand rubs offer an inexpensive alternative to plumbing and sinks but do not completely replace them.

Storage. All medical and office supplies should be stored in an area not visible to patients, with controlled supplies kept in a locked cabinet or drawer. A clean area should be established, and a separate "dirty" area should be designated for the collection of medical waste, needle disposal units, laundry, and temporary storage of reusable items that have not been cleaned, such as instruments and infusion pumps.

Record storage. Space should be allocated for safe and accessible storage of patients' records. If space is at a premium, a rolling, locked cart is an acceptable option.

Staff space. If possible, a quiet, staff-only area should be designated for charting, making phone calls, and reviewing records or resources. Reference books and posted charts or reminders for staff can be kept here out of patients' sight.

Needle and sharps disposal. Each treatment room and the supply room should contain a convenient needle disposal system and waste cans (ideally with a foot pedal and cover) for disposal of both medical and nonmedical waste. The needle disposal units are best kept within arm's reach of the nurse doing vascular access or line care.

Patient education and entertainment. Space selection and design should also consider the needs patients may have for education about OPAT and, at times, for confidential counseling. A television monitor for training, games, or movies may also be helpful and entertaining.

■ *Treatment Rooms*

The number and kind of treatment rooms within a suite will depend primarily on the size and nature of the patient population. A typical mix of individual rooms might be (1) a multipurpose room containing a single bed; (2) several small private rooms, each with a single recliner chair, for infusions; and (3) one group treatment room with three or four recliner chairs for infusions.

Multipurpose Room with Electrically Controlled Bed

This room may be used for examinations, procedures, infusions, rest and comfort, training more than one caregiver, or for children to have more space to move around and play in during their own or a parent's infusion (Figure 10.2). Highly emotional or disruptive patients may be treated here. Acoustic privacy and good lighting are critical. Ideally, daylight should be available, with fluorescent light on dimmers, an adjustable procedure lamp, and a wall-mounted reading lamp by the bed. An otoscope and a sphygmomanometer

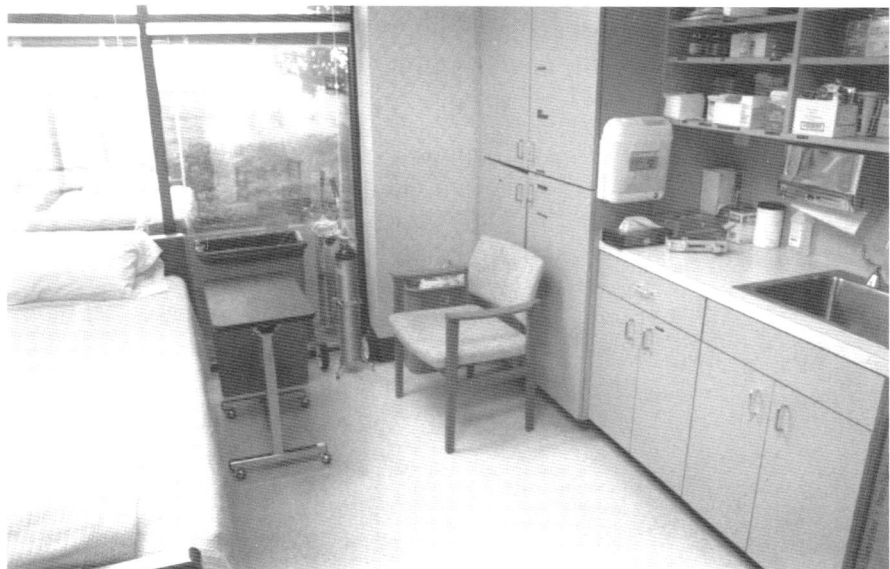

Figure 10.2   *A multipurpose room with an electrically controlled bed is useful for children or highly emotional patients.*

should be mounted on the wall near the bed, along with two additional grounded electrical outlets.

Linoleum is preferable to carpet for floor covering because of potential spills during procedures, such as PICC line insertions. This room definitely should have its own sink and storage for procedure supplies.

Private Room with Recliner

A "living room" look is appropriate here, with carpeting and, if possible, a television set (Figure 10.3). Recliners that do not extend when in the reclining position can be useful if the room is particularly small.

In suites with more than one such room, physicians should consider setting aside one room for the physically handicapped and elderly. The recliner may be replaced with a hardback chair, which can be moved easily to make room for a wheelchair. This room also can be used for brief patient visits, such as an unplanned peripheral catheter restart.

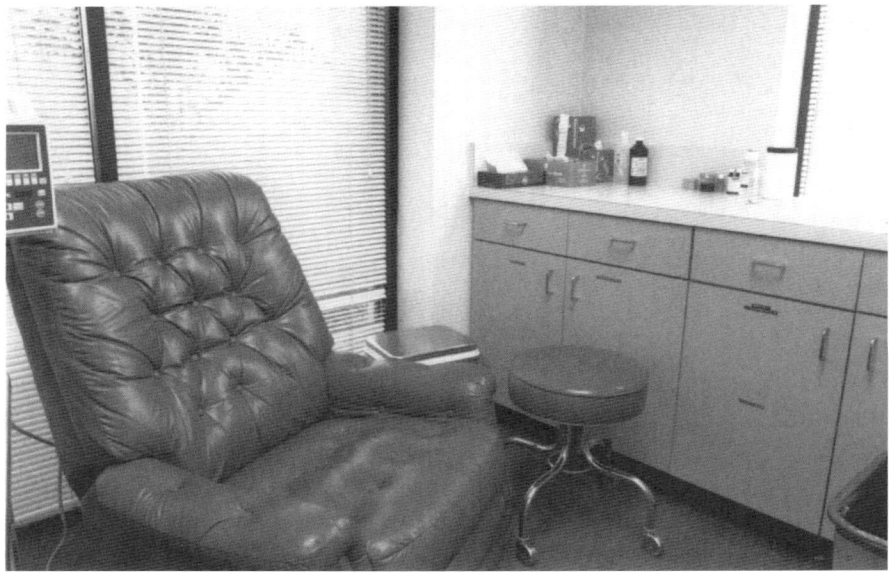

Figure 10.3   *A private room with a comfortable reclining chair, magazines, good reading light, and perhaps carpeting and a small TV can help patients feel relaxed.*

Group Treatment Room

This room should contain a maximum of four recliners, separated by ceiling-hung cubicle curtains. Most patients who are otherwise healthy can be treated here, and many sicker patients actually prefer to have company during infusions.

■ *Nurses' Station*

This area should be centrally located, with a clear view of the infusion rooms. Although a central island accomplishes this, it lacks acoustic privacy for discussions of patient problems. A better arrangement might be to locate the station at the head of a corridor with the rooms off both sides.

■ *Treatment Supply Room*

Located close to the nurses' station, this room should contain a sink, refrigerator, and a counter for the preparation of equipment and supplies. The area should be large enough for two people to work in at the same time. Ideally, this should be a separate room, inaccessible to unsupervised patients or visitors. It should be designated as "clean" and not be used for storage of any "dirty" items.

■ *Staff Room*

This room, which provides a change of atmosphere from the patient care area, can be used for meetings, breaks, and staff education. A secured closet, lockers, or drawers should be available here for storage of staff's personal belongings. Refreshments, food, or coffee may be allowed but pose a risk in regard to infection control.

■ *Reception/Waiting Area*

A reception counter should have a privacy screen and a separate area should be set aside for questions regarding bills. Consider non-invasive, pleasant diversions for both children and adults, such as magazines; washable toys; and potentially, entertainment stations and fish tanks.

■ *Toilets*

No special regulations are applicable here, except those of the Americans with Disabilities Act (ADA). However, toilets should be near the patient care areas and should accommodate an IV pole as well as the patient and a nurse if needed.

■ *Building Regulations*

All local building, health department, ADA, U.S. Occupational Safety and Health Administration, and any other building code requirements must be met. Physicians seeking accreditation by the JCAHO, Community Health Accreditation Program, or the Accreditation Association for Ambulatory Health Care should review the relevant organization's physical plant standards for ambulatory care and/or ambulatory infusion centers when designing hallway size, exits, emergency plans, and infection control features.

Finally, in designing an infusion suite, physicians should involve staff members who will be working in the space. Their perspective and ideas will be valuable in developing a facility that is both functional and attractive. Patients are also a good source for suggestions.

Index

OPAT Handbook/CME Posttest and Evaluation Form

Participation in this educational activity should be completed in approximately 4 hours. **To successfully complete this activity and receive credit, both the Posttest and CME Evaluation Form must be received by AAF-MED no later than August 31, 2007.**

- Read the Statement of Need, Target Audience, and Learning Objectives
- Read *Handbook of Outpatient Parenteral Antimicrobial Therapy for Infectious Diseases* in its entirety
- Complete BOTH the CME Evaluation Form and Posttest. Fax or mail to AAF-MED at the address on page 131. If faxing, be sure to fax both sides of the page.
- A grade of 70% or higher is required to receive credit. A certificate of earned credit will be mailed based on your professional degree, so be sure to complete the profile information on page 129.

For information on applicability and acceptance of continuing education credit for this activity, please consult your professional licensing board.

Once you have completed the Posttest:

- Be sure your profile and contact information is complete and legible
- Be sure you have answered all the questions by circling the letter of the selected answer choice (there is one correct answer per question)
- Tear the Posttest and CME Evaluation Form from the *Handbook of Outpatient Parenteral Antimicrobial Therapy for Infectious Diseases* along the perforation, fold, and place in a standard-size business envelope, stamp, and mail OR fax both sides to 914-703-6435
- Be sure to return your materials before August 31, 2007

Supported by an educational grant from Cubist Pharmaceuticals, Inc.

125

OPAT Handbook/CME Posttest

Name: _____ Date: _____

Complete the following multiple choice questions by circling the letter of the selected answer choice. There is one correct answer per question.

1. Self-administration of OPAT is not possible for patients sent home from the hospital with an IV line in place.
   a. True
   b. False

2. Home infusion companies are usually organized around:
   a. Pharmacy services
   b. Medical care by physicians
   c. Visiting nurse services
   d. All of the above

3. Patients who live alone should never be considered for OPAT.
   a. True
   b. False

4. Patients with endocarditis can be considered for OPAT if they:
   a. Are infected with any of the HACEK group organisms
   b. Have rhythm disturbances
   c. Have left-sided infections with large vegetations
   d. Are not within a short distance of emergency medical care

5. Given the growing resistance of *S. aureus* to methicillin and vancomycin, patients with skin and soft tissue infections should probably not be treated with:
   a. Ceftriaxone
   b. Ertapenem
   c. Daptomycin
   d. None of the above

6. HIV-positive patients who remain immunosuppressed and therefore need prolonged IV therapy with toxic medications for opportunistic infections must always be treated in the hospital.
   a. True
   b. False

7. In a 2005 study, Corwin and associates demonstrated that patients with cellulitis who were assigned to either home or hospital care:
   a. Showed better outcomes with OPAT
   b. Had fewer days on IV and oral antibiotics in the hospital
   c. Did not differ significantly for most primary and outcome measures
   d. Reported greater satisfaction with home care

8. In a recent study of blood sampling from peripherally inserted central venous catheters (PICCs) in children, children whose catheters were used for sampling showed a significantly higher occlusion rate.
   a. Sampling was associated with a significant increase in infection
   b. Investigators concluded that blood sample through PICCs is feasible and effective
   c. None of the above

9. Implanted ports solve some of the problems associated with long-term or intermittent OPAT using tunneled central venous catheters (CVCs) and PICCs, because they:
   a. Require little maintenance between infusions
   b. Are safely concealed beneath the patient's skin
   c. Are impervious to water
   d. All of the above

10. The usual antimicrobial regimen given to OPAT patients does not involve:
    a. Intermittent delivery
    b. Infusion at rates of 50 to 100 ml/h over 30 minutes to 3 hours up to 4x/day
    c. Absolute accuracy and continuity of flow
    d. Infusion of the complete dose within a reasonable period

11. Under Medicare Part B, reimbursable home IV drug therapy includes:
    a. Any antimicrobial
    b. External and implantable pumps
    c. Only prolonged infusions of 8 hours or more
    d. Payment for administration by a nurse on a physician's orders

12. Most major private health insurance policies have some provision for OPAT, but they may also:
    a. Require prior authorization for treatment
    b. Cover outpatient care at a lower percentage of billed charges than those of hospitalization
    c. Cover OPAT charges at a lower percentage if the beneficiary does not use a "preferred provider" contracted with the payer
    d. All of the above

13. Physicians who prescribe OPAT for patients and are, or select, the providers of care should be aware that as "captain of the ship," they:
    a. Must personally supervise the treatment of all patients
    b. May appoint a nurse or pharmacist as primary caregiver as long as they sign the necessary reimbursement forms
    c. Are not liable for the quality of care delivered to patients if they don't deliver it personally
    d. Carry the ultimate responsibility and potential liability for patient care regardless of who actually delivers treatment

14. In *Wickline v State of California*, the physician was held responsible for the loss of a patient's leg from gangrene because:
    a. He discharged the patient too early
    b. The patient was discharged earlier than he advised due to pressure from the HMO, but he should have objected more strenuously
    c. The patient insisted on being discharged and the physician agreed
    d. The patient signed himself out of the hospital against the advice of the physician who should have objected more strenuously

OPAT Handbook/CME Posttest

Name: _____

Degrees and Credentials: _____

Institution: _____

Address 1: _____

Address 2: _____

City/State/Zip Code: _____

Phone: _____

Fax: _____

E-mail: _____

I claim _____ (up to 4) *AMA PRA Category 1 Credits*™   OR

I spent _____ (up to 4) hours in this activity and require a certificate of participation.

Signature: _____   Date: _____

Please sign and date and return with your posttest and evaluation to:

AAF-MED
660 White Plains Road, Suite 535
Tarrytown, NY 10591
Phone (914) 703-6439 Fax (914) 703-6435
Email: info@aafmed.com

Allow 6 weeks for a response.

Were the learning objectives met?

(1) Identify patient candidates for OPAT ☐ Yes ☐ No
from those presenting in the office or
those already hospitalized

(2) Name the infections amenable to OPAT ☐ Yes ☐ No

(3) List the antimicrobial(s) appropriate to
treating specific diseases with OPAT ☐ Yes ☐ No

(4) Define the most appropriate intravenous ☐ Yes ☐ No
catheter for antimicrobial delivery according to individual patient situations and
preferences

(5) Appraise whether a port should be placed, ☐ Yes ☐ No
depending on the patient's condition, treatment situation, and preference; be able to
choose the port that is most appropriate

(6) Describe the infusion device best suited to ☐ Yes ☐ No
the patient's treatment requirements and
preference

(7) Detail a quality measurement program ☐ Yes ☐ No
based on clinical outcomes as well as program structure and process

(8) As a referring physician, define an OPAT ☐ Yes ☐ No
program that will fulfill an individual patient's needs for safe, effective, quality care

   (9) Recognize the legal issues associated   □ Yes   □ No
        with OPAT
  (10) Evaluate reimbursement from Medicare,   □ Yes   □ No
        Medicaid, Blue Cross/Blue Shield
If not, why not? _____

_____

2. This activity received commercial support.
    Acknowledgment of commercial support was
    disclosed at the beginning of the activity.

    The activity was balanced and free from   □ Yes   □ No
    commercial bias.

3. Do you anticipate making changes in your   □ Yes   □ No
    practice as a result of this activity?

Please list any changes _____

_____

4. Overall rating of activity
    □ Excellent   □ Very Good   □ Good   □ Fair   □ Poor

Please complete your evaluation and return it with your credit-claim form to:
AAF-MED
660 White Plains Road, Suite 535
Tarrytown, New York 10591
Phone: (914) 703-6439 Fax: (914) 703-6435
Email: info@aafmed.com